thegoodwebguide

health

thegoodwebguide

health

Jenni Muir

The Good Web Guide Limited • London

First published in Great Britain in 2000 by The Good Web Guide Limited
Broadwall House, 21 Broadwall, London, SE1 9PL

www.thegoodwebguide.co.uk

Email:feedback@thegoodwebguide.co.uk

Original series concept by Steve Bailey

Cover photo © Telegraph Colour Library

10 9 8 7 6 5 4 3 2 1

A catalogue record for this book is available from the British Library.

ISBN 1-903282-08-X

Project Editor Michelle Clare

Design by Myriad Creative Ltd

Printed in Italy at LEGO S.p.A.

contents

the good web guides

The World Wide Web is a vast resource, with millions of sites on every conceivable subject. There are people who have made it their mission to surf the net: cyber-communities have grown, and people have formed relationships and even married on the net.

However, the reality for most people is that they don't have the time or inclination to surf the net for hours on end. Busy people want to use the internet for quick access to information. You don't have to spend hours on the internet looking for answers to your questions and you don't have to be an accomplished net surfer or cyber wizard to get the most out of the web. It can be a quick and useful resource if you are looking for specific information.

The Good Web Guides have been published with this in mind. To give you a head start in your search, our researchers have looked at hundreds of sites and what you will find in the Good Web Guides is a collection of reviews of the best we've found.

The Good Web Guide recommendation is impartial and all the sites have been visited several times. Reviews are focused on the website and what it sets out to do, rather than an endorsement of a company, or their product. A small but beautiful site run by a one-man band may be rated higher than an ambitious but flawed site run by a mighty organisation.

Relevance to the UK-based visitor is also given a high premium: tantalising as it is to read about purchases you can make in California, because of delivery charges, import duties and controls it may not be as useful as a local site.

Our reviewers considered a number of questions when reviewing the sites, such as: How quickly do the sites and individual pages download? Can you move around the site easily and get back to where you started, and do the links work? Is the information up to date and accurate? And is the site pleasing to the eye and easy to read? More importantly, we also asked whether the site has something distinctive to offer, whether it be entertainment, inspiration or pure information. On the basis of the answers to these questions sites are given ratings out of five. As we aim only to include sites that we feel are of serious interest, there are very few low-rated sites.

Bear in mind that the collection of reviews you see here are just a snapshot of the sites at a particular time. The process of choosing and writing about sites is rather like painting the Forth Bridge: as each section appears complete, new sites are launched and others are modified. When you've registered at the Good Web Guide site (see p. 10 for further details) you can check out the reviews of new sites and updates of existing ones, or even have them emailed to you. By using the cd rom at the back of the book or registering at our site, you'll find hot links to all the sites listed, so you can just click and go without needing to type the addresses accurately into your browser.

As this is the first edition of the Good Web Guide, all our sites have been reviewed by the author and research team, but we'd like to know what you think. Contact us via the website or email feedback@thegoodwebguide.co.uk. You are welcome to recommend sites, quibble about the ratings, point out changes and inaccuracies or suggest new features to assess.

You can find us at www.thegoodwebguide.co.uk

user key

 £   Subscription

 R   Registration required

    Secure online ordering

 UK   Country of origin

introduction

Heard of option paralysis? It's not a disease, although it can be rather debilitating. It's a term used to describe those occasions when you have so many good possibilities in front of you that you just can't choose. If you have not experienced it before, you may well do now. The internet has a mind-boggling number of health sites and many of them are very good.

There is an oft-quoted statistic (though no one in the business is quite sure where it came from) that health is the most popular subject on the internet after pornography. Whether you want to know more about specific diseases, psychological conditions, surgery, leading a healthy life, alternatives to drug therapy, natural ways to prevent or treat illness, or indeed relationships and sexual health, the internet is a wonderful resource. It can help you lose weight, put weight on, find a health club, find a doctor, dentist or therapist, shop for food, vitamins and gym clothes, meet fellow sufferers, fellow enthusiasts or, indeed, fellows.

But with all this information and opportunity we need to be able to sort the good from the less good and the bad. In schools these days children are taught to assess the mass of information presented to them factually on the internet and other media; those of us adults who have not learned these skills need to acquire them. This guide should prove some help, particularly for anyone a little uncomfortable using the internet. We have selected for you more than 120 of the very best and most useful health sites and provide links straight to them so you do not need to use search engines. That means no more typing in 'thrush' to be presented with a list of 431 documents about songbirds of the Turdinae family, inflamations common to frogs and horses, the homepage of the Thrush family in south west Dakota, or a new album called Thrush Hour by an obscure Norwegian heavy metal band.

One of the hardest tasks is keeping up to date with things on the internet because 'things are changing so fast'. We post regular updates and new reviews on our own website at www.thegoodwebguide.co.uk and hope you'll refer to them. Rest assured, however, that our overwhelming experience is that, for the most part, the best sites are those that have been established the longest. They are the ones with the most content and facilities, and the staff have had time to see what works and what doesn't in terms of writing style, design and ease of use. Please enjoy surfing, and don't hesitate to send us your comments so that they may be included in the next edition.

Jenni Muir, July 2000

acknowledgements

This guide could not have been put together without the assistance of Claire Clifton and Ian Fenn who have contributed their expert opinions and research skills, particularly in relation to the chapters on shopping and men's health. Marina Vokos has been very helpful in promoting the books, full of ideas and enthusiasm. Thanks also to friends and colleagues Martin Bumpsteed, Mike Doxey and Vanessa Courtier, all the people who responded so positively to the first book, and everyone at The Good Web Guides, especially Michelle and Elaine who have proved so patient and cooperative.

How to use your CD

When we've whetted your appetite for the sites reviewed in this book, we can help you to visit them quickly and easily. By registering on thegoodwebguide site, you will be able to use the hotlinks to all the sites listed, so you just click and go. You can also read the latest versions of reviews and see what we think of new sites that have been launched since the book went to press. If you wish, you can even have the updates emailed to you.

INSTALLATION INSTRUCTIONS FOR PC USERS

Insert the CD enclosed with this book into your CD drive of your PC. A welcome screen will appear with two buttons:

The goodwebguide button To register your purchase of a Good Web Guide book and to receive free updates of the reviews in the book and reviews of the latest sites, click on this button. When you've registered you can click straight through to any of the sites listed. You must have an internet connection to do this. If you are not already signed up with an internet service, you will need to install the LineOne software first.

If you click on the goodwebguide button you will be taken to a registration page where you will be asked to confirm which title in the series you have bought and to register your details. You then have free access to the updates of the website reviews in this book and to new reviews. You will also have access to the rest of the goodwebguide website.

LineOne button If you would like access to the internet you can click on this button to install LineOne's free ISP (internet service provider) software. You will need a modem to have internet access. If you already have an internet connection (ISP) you can still install LineOne as an alternative provider.

A To join LineOne just click on the LineOne button. When the first screen appears you have a choice: If you are a new user and wish to load Internet Explorer 5 as your browser, select 'Join Now'. On the next screen, select 'Go!' and you will be taken to the Microsoft installation process.

B To join immediately, without installing a browser, click 'Join Now' and then choose 'custom' to go straight to registration.

From the 'Welcome to LineOne' screen, click 'Go' and follow the on-screen instructions.

MAC USERS

This CD is not suitable for Apple Macintosh computers. For Free LineOne Mac Software call free on 0800 111 210.

RETURNING TO THE GOOD WEB GUIDE

Once you've connected to the internet, you can either type www.thegoodwebguide.co.uk into your browser to go directly to our website, or re-insert your CD and click on the goodwebguide button.

SUPPORT
If you have any problems call the LineOne support number.
CALL 0906 30 20 100
(calls may be monitored or recorded for training purposes) 24 hours, 365 days a year. Calls charged at 50p/minute or email support@lineone.net for free support.

Other great titles in thegoodwebguide series:

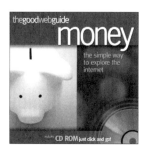

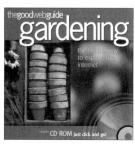

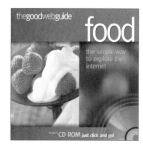

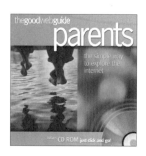

Money	Gardening	Food	Parents
ISBN 1-903282-02-0	ISBN 1-903282-00-4	ISBN 1-903282-01-2	ISBN 1-903282-03-9

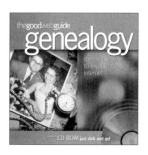

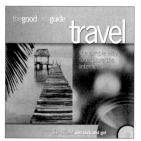

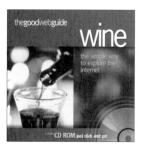

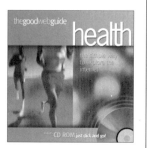

Genealogy	Travel	Wine	Health
ISBN 1-903282-06-3	ISBN 1-903282-05-5	ISBN 1-903282-04-7	ISBN 1-903282-08-X

Chapter 1

general medical sites

Anyone who has sat for hours in a GP's waiting room only to be hurried out of the office after a few minutes before the problem was satisfactorily dealt with can probably understand the attraction of online health consultations. Then there's all those occasions when you feel quite under the weather but worry that it's not a problem serious enough to be bothering a busy doctor with. Perhaps you just need a repeat prescription and it seems silly to have to wait all that time just to walk out with a bit of paper.

No one would argue that our health system needs to be and could be better, and the internet could play an advantageous role. The British government has already recognised this and we now have NHS Direct, a site that received 1.5 million hits on the first day of its launch. Forward-thinking doctors have also been acting on their own initiative. For example, London-based Dr Julian Eden, who has for some years acted as doctor via email to patients of his on diving and mountaineering expeditions,

has launched e-med.co.uk, a site that offers online and telephone consultations. The basic fee is £15 per consultation, plus an initial joining charge of £20. If after discussing the problem he feels a face-to-face appointment is necessary, you need to visit the surgery and for that meeting will be charged £40 - it's also therefore rather important that you live or work nearby. There are some people who will never find such an arrangement satisfactory; others, especially busy professionals, think it brilliant.

Initial concerns about online consultations centred on the fact that they can't fully replace meeting with your doctor face to face, but as Eden's excellent model demonstrates, we can have it both ways - prescriptions emailed to a handy chemist when that's all that's required, or seeing the doctor in person when he needs to investigate closely. And, thanks to webcam, it won't be long before it's normal for our doctors to see us without being in the same room.

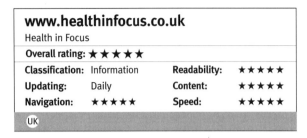

www.healthinfocus.co.uk

Health in Focus

Overall rating: ★ ★ ★ ★ ★			
Classification:	Information	Readability:	★ ★ ★ ★ ★
Updating:	Daily	Content:	★ ★ ★ ★ ★
Navigation:	★ ★ ★ ★ ★	Speed:	★ ★ ★ ★ ★

UK

Accessibility, trustworthiness and unbiased content are the hallmarks of this site, which aims to provide British people with clear and accurate healthcare and medical information. Certainly there is a need for sites to focus on what is available to UK consumers and what is not. As Health in Focus highlights in its background information, many doctors complain that the internet has given patients unrealistic expectations of what they can expect in terms of treatment, and have been disappointed to discover that the experimental 'wonder drugs' discussed on US websites cannot be prescribed in the UK. Health in Focus is part of the publishing company Medicom International Ltd. Funded by educational sponsorships, it is written by healthcare professionals, checked and edited by UK doctors, and approved by patient support groups.

The cleanly designed homepage lacks the gimmicky aspects of more commercial medical sites and sets the serious tone. Content is organised into three columns, the keyword search facility being top centre with a pull-down, quick-find menu top right. News items and weekly features are listed down the left column of the screen. Keep scrolling down the long page for more options. There is also a navigation strip at the top of the screen, offering general reference material.

SPECIAL FEATURES

News Focus Health news is updated Monday to Friday and is largely a round-up of newspaper reports from leading titles such as The Times and Daily Telegraph.

Chat Focus is run in conjunction with the women's channel of msn.co.uk and features guests from specialist associations in a wide variety of conditions, including the British Diabetic Association, the Arthritis Research Campaign, and more. Forthcoming chat sessions and details of how to join in, or how to find further information on the subject, are highlighted. You can also access the archive of previous chats, which includes several conditions: Parkinson's, cot death, breast cancer, mental health, epilepsy, and many more.

Clinical Focus Self-care for sinusitis was being featured on our last visit, but beneath the introductory paragraph was a link to the site's full list of clinical articles. The self-care section is excellent. It answers key questions, such as what the condition is, how to know when you have it, what you can do immediately to make it better, what you can do to avoid it, what treatments can be bought without prescription and when you need to see a doctor. The summary rounds up the most important action to take and invites feedback on the article. At the side of the page are links to pages on frequently asked questions, related conditions, what to do before and after you see a GP, support contacts and helpful websites for each condition, plus the facility to read about other visitors' experiences with the condition. Where new research has been done on the condition, its diagnosis and therapies, Health in Focus offers separate pages with unbiased analysis of the findings. At the top of each article is the name of the writer and the professional doctor who edited it – very reassuring.

Supporter Focus A couple of support and information groups are featured at a time. Our last visit saw the National Osteoporosis Society receiving attention as it was National Osteoporosis Month, as well as the National Eczema Society.

Celebrity Chat Focus   Do you really want to know what a soap star thinks about health issues? This section, which is not as silly as it first seems, was launched just before we went to press. It is inspired not so much by the celebrities but by the plots of their television shows, such as EastEnders' Jackie Owen's struggles with premenstrual syndrome. The soaps can provide a good public service by highlighting particular health issues and diseases, and they increasingly handle such story lines responsibly by providing helplines and information sheets on various conditions, as well as promoting awareness of them.

Men's Health Focus   This content is repurposed from Men's Health Magazine (see p. 150). A question from the latest issue is generally featured, with links to other Q&As, plus a list of featured articles and letters to the editor. Our last visit saw a discussion of the problem of developing pimples on the chest after a sweaty workout.

Alternative Health Focus contains articles on natural health and remedies, supplied by Think Natural.com (see p. 128).

Health Tips Focus features articles by Dr Jeremy Sims, a GP, on preventing various conditions, with one highlighted weekly and the option to browse the archive. It's good on women's health issues, such as endometriosis, fibroids, agnus castus, cystitis, menstrual cramps and subjects such as diet, fitness and nutrition. The cross-referencing to other relevant sections of the site is useful and well done.

Women's Health Focus is produced in association with the msn.co.uk women's health channel. The section is divided into two parts: a list of fact sheets (basically the self-care articles described under Clinical Focus) and the msn.co.uk discussion features.

Discussion Forums   Allergies, coronary heart disease and multiple sclerosis are the suggested topics here, and you are invited to contribute your own ideas as well as respond to postings from others. They did not seem particularly well attended during our reviewing process, but did offer some interesting reading, plus useful links.

Quick Browse   Positioned towards the bottom of the homepage, this offers a substantial list of conditions to click on for further information.

Links   Embarrassing Problems, Care4Free, Scoot, Bupa, Amazon.co.uk, NHS Direct, to sites with Health in Focus-approved information, plus links to external sites with medical reference databases.

OTHER FEATURES

Glossary, health events focus.

A fine site that works hard to be responsible in the way it disseminates information; as they say, their aim is to be 'transparent' in their practices, as well as providers of high quality editorial, uninfluenced by advertisers. We think the site is excellent, but believe it would be enhanced by dropping the repurposed content from companies such as Think Natural and Men's Health and replacing it with original material.

www.mayohealth.org
Mayo Clinic Health Oasis

Overall rating: ★ ★ ★ ★ ★			
Classification:	Information	**Readability:**	★ ★ ★ ★ ★
Updating:	On weekdays	**Content:**	★ ★ ★ ★ ★
Navigation:	★ ★ ★ ★ ★	**Speed:**	★ ★ ★ ★ ★

US

The Mayo Clinic is a non-profit organisation, over 100 years old, and world-famous for its medical expertise. Its traditional philosophy of 'cooperative science' – clinical doctors and specialists working in conjunction with scientists – means that the organisation often makes the discoveries in the news rather than following them, so this site is a must for those who want to be on the leading edge of health information. The site is directed by a large team of Mayo physicians, scientists, writers and educators, with the aim of providing health education to Mayo patients and the general public. All articles are dated, so you can tell when they were placed on the site, and those over three years old are reviewed for continuing accuracy. The homepage is very clean in design and easy to navigate; you simply click on the subject that interests you.

SPECIAL FEATURES

New on Oasis incorporates the latest questions answered by the Mayo consultants, including physicians and dietitians, plus articles featuring case studies and cures from disease.

Allergy & Asthma Like all the condition categories or 'centers' featured on the site, this is broken down into several sections including latest headlines, Ask the Mayo Physician, quizzes, a glossary, links and a library of reference articles. The headlines may be gleaned from other sections, such as a quiz in hayfever season, or a new and interesting query from a site visitor, or a news story from the Headline Watch section. At the base of stories are links to other relevant articles in the site's library.

Alzheimer's While the statistics provided are for the US, this section still provides sobering thought. One in ten families has a relative with Alzheimer's disease, and of the four million people who have it, 70 per cent live at home and require care from family members. One excellent feature in this section suggests ways in which the rest of us can give support to these caregivers, 80 per cent of whom report high levels of stress and stress-related illness, and considers why we pull away. Other typical coverage in this section incorporates dementia and memory loss, new treatments, case studies and coping with the end stages of the disease.

Arthritis Lifestyle issues are strong in this channel, such as travelling when you suffer from arthritis and how to cope with arthritis at work. The title is a little misleading, as you will also find information on conditions such as bunions. The useful Treatments section provides information on medications and surgery, but also complementary and alternative treatments and advice on self-care.

Cancer Our last visit saw the Mayo Clinic leading the way in research, having found a means of locating cancer using radioactively modified vitamin B12. A case study of one patient who was able to avoid masectomy thanks to the development was featured, along with a thorough but easy-to-understand explanation of the process, the background research and its potential (including the revelation that the Mayo Clinic is also researching ways in which B12 may be used to treat cancer in future). More news included a warning that some dietary supplements containing a particular Chinese herb can cause kidney failure and urinary system cancer. In general, however, we were disappointed by the lack of coverage of complementary therapies in this section, although amongst the library features were stories such as 'meat and breast cancer – charring, frying increase risk' and dietary guidelines from the American cancer society. The library is organised by types of cancer, plus a prevention section.

Digestive is a broad-reaching section, incorporating information on ulcers, the appendix, constipation, diarrhoea, coeliac disease, gallstones, heartburn, indigestion, diverticulosis, irritable bowel syndrome, liver disease, the pancreas, and more. Amongst the interesting questions posed by site visitors was news that some calcium supplements can cause constipation, and what should be done in these cases.

Heart also incorporates some information on strokes, and emphasises that incidence of both can be dramatically reduced by an increase in activity levels. There is a fascinating story here of a Mayo Clinic doctor with a special interest in researching cardiovascular disease, who suffered a heart attack after being given a clean bill of health from his own doctor only four weeks earlier. This gives a particular authority and poignancy to his advice on the subject.

Medicine You can enter a drug name into the search facility in this channel to find out more about it. There is also advice on the correct usage of medicines, whether prescription or over-the-counter. Amongst the headlines on our last visit was a warning about antibiotics from the World Health Organisation, which reports that drug-resistant infections in both wealthy and developing nations threaten to make once-treatable diseases incurable.

Nutrition In addition to Ask the Dietician, features and quizzes, this channel offers the virtual cookbook, inviting visitors to send in their recipes for a 'healthy makeover'. Recipes are categorised by type of dish, plus a new recipe section highlighting latest additions; the measurements and cookery language are American but they are easy to understand.

Mayo Sports Medicine is subtitled Fitness and Appearance. Here is a library on articles covering medical and physiotherapy conditions, such as ankle sprain rehabilitation, plus lifestyle issues such as exercising as we age ('how to get off the sidelines and back in the game') and obesity ('weight control – what works and why'). In addition, some features are based on avoiding injury in specific sports including golf, snowboarding and mountain biking. There is also an interactive exercise tipsheet. Scroll down beneath this section for 'appearance' issues, such as benign skin markings, body image, body piercing, liposuction and facelifts, acne and wrinkles.

Links Many to support organisations and associations associated with specific conditions.

OTHER FEATURES

Today's Feature, Headline Watch with archive, separate channels for men, women and children's health.

The Mayo Clinic is a must-see for anyone interested in medical health issues, and is a definite favourite of ours amongst the big medical sites.

www.medicdirect.co.uk
Medic Direct

Overall rating: ★ ★ ★ ★			
Classification:	Information	**Readability:**	★ ★ ★ ★
Updating:	Varies	**Content:**	★ ★ ★ ★
Navigation:	★ ★ ★ ★ ★	**Speed:**	★ ★ ★ ★

UK

Its claim to be 'the only interactive website hosted by leading UK medical consultants providing comprehensive health information online' is stretching the point, but it is difficult not to be immediately impressed by this slickly designed and comprehensive resource. The long list of doctors who write and own the site may not include any well-known names, but there is a tremendous collection of qualifications and prestige positions. David Morgan, a consultant ear, nose and throat surgeon, decided to set it up when he found it difficult to track down reliable health information on the internet following his father's stroke.

The attractive homepage, which is designed to look like an open notebook, is very easy to navigate: the key information channels are listed at the centre of the page, with official information, links and other administrative departments in a menu panel down the left-hand side of the screen. You can search the site by keyword from the facility on the homepage. There are also buttons for news and videos pages.

SPECIAL FEATURES

News is updated frequently, but not daily, and covers a variety of health issues, including research findings and campaigns. The brief articles are well written though not referenced or cross-referred, which other sites make a point of doing. This smacks of arrogance – you are expected to take their word for it – but the lack of detail and big words makes the information easy to understand.

Clinics Click here and you will be offered a list of 23 general conditions, including allergies, brain and spinal disorders, elderly medicine, pregnancy, sports injuries and skin conditions. Choose one and more specific problems or situations will be listed on the next page. The length and helpfulness of these articles vary. Where over-the-counter remedies can help a problem, specific products are recommended. Using this section does require you to know already what is wrong with you.

Diseases is another means of presenting the information above. It offers an image of the body with labels pointing to its various systems. Click on the one you want and you are taken through to a list of possible conditions. We found it easier to find the information we were looking for here, although this cannot always be the case, as many of the conditions listed are things you will never have heard of.

Operations works as the diseases section – you click on the system of the body you are looking for information about. Again, it's not foolproof. To look up a nasal operation you actually need to click on the chest for respiratory system. The information, however, is useful. It explains briefly how the operation is performed, how long it takes, time in hospital required, risks and complications, outcomes and post-operative discomfort, and time off work. Some of the operations offer video footage.

Tests covers antenatal, blood, endoscopy, heart, lungs, urine, X-rays and special tests such as lumbar punctures and liver biopsies. This information seeks to answer common questions such as 'what are they for?' and 'what do they mean?'. It also explains the technique and, where appropriate, has pictures.

Minor Ailments We were surprised to be presented with a diagram of a house and garden when clicking on this channel. Apparently minor ailments occur in particular rooms, which will be news to anyone with a sore throat that seems to go everywhere with you. Enough injuries are listed under the bedroom to keep you awake all night, including athlete's foot, bad breath, carbon monoxide poisoning, foreign bodies in the nose, head lice and scabies, nose bleed, unconsciousness and, of course, headaches. Design affectations aside, this channel would be more appropriate if it emphasised injuries and illnesses that happen in various places: since when are carbon monoxide poisoning and electrocution minor ailments?

Self Examination is 'your guide to early diagnosis in the home'. Here you will find downloadable videos of conducting breast and testicular examinations, advice on how to check your moles for early signs of skin cancer, and the glass test for detecting the early signs of meningitis. A very useful section.

Lifestyle is primarily divided into the 'seven ages of man' and offers information on diet, exercise and screening for each stage, though the 'future parents' stage is for pregnant women. The choice here of medieval stained glass images to illustrate is highly appropriate because some of the thinking behind the information presented is indeed from the Dark Ages. It's no wonder that so many people do not find the medical profession a satisfactory point of reference when it comes to being and staying well. Vegetarianism and zen macrobiotics are presented as 'common food fads which may lead to serious problems'. Other topics include alcohol, smoking and stress-saving strategies. The information given is very basic. Also here is a weekly, magazine-style column from sports writer Mel Webb.

Student Health covers alcohol, drugs, smoking, sex (including gay), fitness and finances (with links to student banks), all presented with a jazzy typeface for 'yoof' appeal. Why, however, do they think that only students would be interested in the impact of mobile phones on health? Do they use them more than the rest of us? We think not...

Links to support groups and other organisations dealing with health-related matters. The links database has to be searched by keyword.

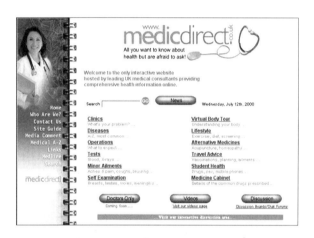

OTHER FEATURES

Virtual Body Tour, Alternative Medicines, Travel Advice, medicine cabinet, medical A-Z, GP/medical practitioner information and discussion services, media comment.

Although the design elements are more pretentious than useful, this is a fine site if you are looking for information on medical conditions and things that you may experience in the doctor's surgery or hospital. It can give you the basics of healthy living advice, but it is patronising in tone and not at the forefront of nutrition thinking.

www.netdoctor.co.uk			
Net Doctor			
Overall rating: ★ ★ ★ ★			
Classification: Information		**Readability:**	★ ★ ★ ★ ★
Updating: Daily		**Content:**	★ ★ ★ ★ ★
Navigation: ★ ★ ★ ★ ★		**Speed:**	★ ★ ★
UK			

According to the company background information, over 250 British and other European doctors and health care professionals provide content for this medical site. Most recognisable amongst the contributors are Dr Hilary Jones, the GP of GMTV, and author Dr Gillian Rice, but the site's senior UK Medical Director is Dr Dan Rutherford. Net Doctor claims: 'As a matter of policy our doctors, writers and editors are not allowed to be influenced by or answerable to our sponsors or advertisers. We follow the same standards of practice as the leading medical journals.' The company believes that, in the future, most patients will seek out critical health information on the internet, and aims to 'break down the medical language barrier' between doctor and patient. However, as the disclaimer highlights in red: 'The material presented in Net Doctor is in no way intended to replace professional medical care or attention by a qualified practitioner... The material on NetDoctor.co.uk cannot and should not be used as a basis for diagnosis or choice of treatment.' That is, it's for information purposes only.

At the top of the homepage is a box for searching the site by keyword. Below are listed categories of reference and interactive and feature material, with news and timely features listed in the panel down the right of the screen; if you have a small screen, you may find some pages difficult to read as they are designed a little too wide. The

site has three main channels: Encyclopedia, Interactive and Special Features.

SPECIAL FEATURES

Diseases and Conditions Clicking here takes you to a search page that allows you to find information by the first letter of the medical condition you want to know about, or to type in a keyword. They believe they have the most extensive health information on the web but, if you can't find what you're looking for, they invite you to email Dr Dan Rutherford direct to tell him what's missing.

Health Advice is part of the encyclopedia channel. It offers general advice on health and well-being, and is broken down into broad, popular categories including allergies, children's health, senior citizens, minor injuries, safety and first aid, and so on. Curiously, the only entry under men's health is 'male hair loss' – a pretty poor showing given the extraordinary amount of coverage given to children's health, childbirth and similar parenting subjects. Nevertheless, we found some good, practical self-help tips on certain subjects that could relieve a lot of non-life-threatening suffering – for example, foods and drinks to avoid, whether or not to lie down, how to prop oneself up with a pillow and, of course, whether to consult a doctor. At the end of these pages is an extensive list of links to related chapters on the site and contact details of support groups.

Medicines offers an alphabetical or keyword search of particular products. Click on the one you want to know more about and an information sheet will come up stating its main use, active ingredient and manufacturer. Beneath this, questions such as 'how does it work?' and 'what it is used for?' are answered, and the key warnings about the product are supplied, such as its side effects, circumstances in which it should be used with caution or not at all, what it cannot be taken in conjunction with and warnings given on the label. This is particularly useful when you are on long-term medication and develop a more transient problem, such as a cold or flu – it may be dangerous to take certain remedies for the latter while on the former.

Topic Overview is the section to go to when you're not sure what you're looking for. Here you can look up broad subject categories such as 'accidents and sports injuries', 'eyes', 'vaccinations', 'heart, blood and circulation', 'men's diseases', and so on. You will then be taken to more specific listings of pages from other sections of the site, broken down into diseases, health advice, discussion, ask the doctor and test yourself.

News is available on a daily basis on the site, and you can sign up to have it delivered free by email. The information is archived, too, so that you can search for stories by date or keyword. Also here is daily international health news from Reuters bureau.

Test Yourself Although this section was earmarked for expansion as we went to press, there were several questionnaires here to help you establish the risk of developing, or likelihood of having, certain medical conditions. Topics covered included asthma, depression, diabetes, smoking, alcohol, weight problems, prostate cancer and pregnancy. They included the silly 'what day of the week were you born?', the commonsense 'are you an apple or a pear?', the practical 'monitor your pregnancy week by week' and the revealing 'could you be depressed?'

Discuss features nearly 50 topics of discussion, of which 'men's problems' and 'women's problems' seem to be the most popular. Pregnancy, depression, skin problems, and stomach and digestion problems are also well attended. We liked the fact that postings received within the last 24 hours were indicated by bold numbers and that there is an option to view the last 50 postings. As they state, you need to bear in mind that the opinions expressed on these forums are those of the general public and not the site's medical team.

Ask the Doctor offers the opportunity to post questions to the site's experts, and read previous answers, which go on to form a significant proportion of the site's reference material. The answers can be browsed by category or the ten latest additions to the site. However, comparatively few questions are answered, given the number Net Doctor receives, and they do their best to talk you out of posting a question before they let you submit one – so, like many other sites on the net, the facility to ask the experts is a bit of a swizz.

Links to advertisers, which include goodandgreen.com and allcures.com.

OTHER FEATURES

Sex & Relationships, Children, Pregnancy & Childbirth, Examinations, Special Reports, Live Chat, Find a Health Service, Support Groups, Code of Ethics.

It is pleasing to have a good large British medical site, although it lacks the depth of the long-established American sites, such as Mayo Clinic Health Oasis (see p. 16). There is a bias towards sex and relationships, pregnancy and children's health, as opposed to debilitating and life-threatening diseases, which may reflect the British population's supposed preoccupations.

www.nhsdirect.nhs.uk
NHS Direct Online

Overall rating: ★ ★ ★ ★ ★			
Classification:	Homepage	**Readability:**	★ ★ ★ ★ ★
Updating:	Monthly	**Content:**	★ ★ ★ ★ ★
Navigation:	★ ★ ★ ★ ★	**Speed:**	★ ★ ★ ★ ★

UK

NHS Direct is a 24-hour telephone helpline led by National Health Service nurses that offers information and advice to patients and the general public. The online service, while also an information resource, is different in that it does not offer 'consultations'. Instead, its aim is to sift through the 100,000+ health-related sites on the internet and recommend those that offer good quality information to the public. It is an initiative that has already proved effective in America through the US government's healthfinder.gov and medlineplus (www.nlm.nih.gov/medlineplus) sites.

The homepage is very easy to navigate, with a menu strip across the top of the screen and an explanation of the contents in each section below. Pages on the site are kept short, so this site is easy to use if you have a small screen.

SPECIAL FEATURES

Health Features includes a monthly magazine with a different focus in each 'issue'. On our most recent visit, travel health was in the spotlight, and links were provided to relevant sites. Also here is a monthly online chat – the heart and cancer were typical topics of discussion and were hosted by specialist doctors in the field. Behind the Scenes at NHS Direct offers some insight into the workings of the organisation, such as the fact that the service is most popular in holiday destinations because people are away from their regular doctors. The Health in the News section is derived from sources such as the BBC, GMTV, and the Guardian. As we went to press, the section titled Advice from the Chief Medical Officer, Liam Donaldson, had not been updated for a few months – it was article- and comment-led rather than giving direct advice on health problems, and contained an article encouraging people who are trying to stop smoking to continue trying to quit.

Healthy Living is produced by the Health Education Authority and focuses on achievable lifestyle changes to help you live longer, feel (and look) better and reduce your chances of falling ill. While it covers the usual lifestyle issues, such as diet and nutrition, exercise, alcohol and cigarette consumption, stress, and so on, it also impressively raises the issues of factors outside the individual's control, such as poverty, social exclusion, housing, education, employment and the environment. It also links you to information on the UK government's health strategy: 'Saving Lives: Our Healthier Nation'. Click in the menu panel down the side for access to general advice on improving your health (including your teeth), or for tips on reducing the risk of a long list of conditions including various cancers, depression, heart disease, HIV and AIDS, osteoporosis, sexually transmitted diseases, and accidents. Although the information and advice here is concise, it is also very good and well cross-referenced, where appropriate, to other tips from the NHS.

Healthcare Guide aims to be a 'first step' to help you decide the best course of action when a common health problem arises. It offers a body key as a means of assessing what symptoms you or the sufferer may have, then asks a series of questions in order to establish what advice and action you need to follow, whether that is self-care, calling NHS Direct or dialling 999. Where the guide suggests self-care, it tells you what to do, what you can buy from a chemist that may help, and organisations to contact for further advice. There is also a glossary of conditions, a guide to stocking a simple medicine chest for the home, a section titled 'how do I know if my baby is ill?', and another on how to identify an emergency. This may sound superfluous, but reports reveal that people dial 999 for astonishingly trivial matters.

A-Z Guide to the NHS 'Finding your way around the National Health Service can be difficult, particularly at a time when you may be ill or worried.' When services are also provided by voluntary agencies and social services, the picture is more clouded. This section, derived from the 1991 Patient's Charter, seeks to demystify the organisation and help you get more out of it. The database includes information about how the NHS is funded and structured, who does what, how to access services when you need them, how to complain and make suggestions, and more.

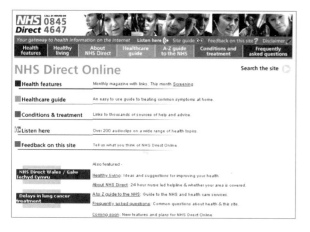

Conditions and Treatment There are three means of searching this section: by keyword, text search or clicking on the body map, which is a cyber-style drawing that has the main body parts labelled from head to feet. Within each body part, several conditions are covered. For example, in

the Upper Body you can read information relating to ailments of the chest, lungs and heart; the Abdomen offers a long list, from alpha one antitrypsin deficiency to worms.

Frequently Asked Questions offers a variety of concise answers to what are, apparently, very common questions about health conditions and lifestyle choices and, in a separate section, the NHS. It also suggests articles and links for further information.

Listen Here offers more than 200 audioclips, ranging from three to ten minutes, on a very wide range of health topics. Real Audio is required to hear them and, if you don't have a recent browser, this can be downloaded by clicking on the link supplied. Some pieces of information are available in Asian languages, including Urdu and Bengali. The section is constantly updated with new material.

Links to thousands of sources of help, advice and articles, importantly the National Electronic Library for Health (NeLH), but also to things as commercial as Lonely Planet and Rough Guide for tips on travel health.

This is an excellent service, and impressively simple to use and understand; a lot of thought has clearly gone into making it accessible and useful for all. Although conservative and conventional in its approach to treatments, it is comforting that the information has NHS approval or backing, and the editorial offers plenty of preventative health advice as well as instructions for what to do when someone has already fallen ill.

www.onhealth.com			
On Health			
Overall rating: ★ ★ ★ ★			
Classification:	Information	**Readability:**	★ ★ ★ ★ ★
Updating:	Daily	**Content:**	★ ★ ★ ★ ★
Navigation:	★ ★ ★ ★ ★	**Speed:**	★ ★ ★
US			

On Health is chattier in style than its large American counterparts Web MD and Mayo Clinic, and more like a health magazine than a serious reference site. That doesn't mean its information is less credible; it's merely delivered in a friendlier fashion. Some of the material – healthy eating features, for example – is featured in more than one section, which means you need not aim to read the whole site.

The homepage is particularly easy to navigate: simply choose your desired channel from the menu panel down the left-hand side of the screen.

SPECIAL FEATURES

Diseases & Conditions Our last visit saw this channel leading with a feature titled 'Frequently Unasked Questions', which emphasised the importance of speaking to one's doctor about embarrassing problems. Plenty of other articles are included in this section and on the right of the screen there is an alphabetical reference guide to conditions. There is a section for Diseases and Conditions News, and discussion boards on diabetes, cancers, and aches and pains are highlighted. Dr Robert Jandl, one of the channel's key contributors, advocates Listening to Your Body on the discussion board of the same name. He answers questions from site visitors in-depth, and even quite lengthy answers are easy to read thanks to the site's excellent design.

Women Although there is an element of beauty coverage in this section, with pages on skin maintenance and dandruff, there is plenty of medical information, too, such as question and answer 'clinics' on hormone replacement therapy and heart disease in women, breast cancer pages, a case study and discussion of gastric bypass surgery and the implications of amenorrhoea (loss of periods). Features are cross-referenced to related articles and the encyclopedia sections.

Family Dr Kathi J Kemper is the holistic paediatrician contributing to this channel, and on our last visit was recommending safe natural treatments for dry skin in children (forget vitamin E and use olive oil was the advice she offered). It's not all about children, however: there's advice here on family relationships, and Dr Walter Bortz offers tips on active aging.

Baby Typical content in this channel is the benefits of infant massage, arguments for and against vaccination, why you should take a holiday before the baby is born, teenage pregnancy, myths about pregnancy and fertility, and understanding ectopic pregnancy. There are clinics in this channel on children's growth problems, and cold and flu, plus a reference section on baby conditions and 'baby' news headlines, some of which is supplied by major news bureaux.

Alternative Dr James Dillard is the celebrity practitioner of this channel. On our last visit he was discussing whether chocolate was a good medicine or an addictive treat, and extolling the virtues of tai chi for stress reduction. Also here was advice on finding a good massage therapist, discussion boards on anxiety and fibromyalgia, a quiz to test your knowledge about common medicinal herbs, advice on relieving postpartum breast engorgement, and pages on healing prayer, cancer-fighting foods and irritable bowel syndrome. A wide brief indeed, and, if you get confused, there's always the Understanding Alternatives section, which aims to reveal 'how to tell homeopathy from naturopathy, rolfing from reiki'.

Lifestyle   High-profile 'life coach' Cheryl Richardson was headlining this channel on our last visit with a feature about taking the symptoms of stress seriously. She is but one of several contributors to this channel, which seems to be something of a mish-mash of features lifted from the others, but makes good reading in its own right. Sex matters are covered here by Louanne Cole Weston PhD, a certified sex therapist and family counsellor, and several interesting features and discussions were included in her archive. A test was offered called 'What's Draining You?' and offered remedies to 'plug the drain'. Amongst the subjects discussed in the clinics were stress management, when to see a therapist, and coping with seasonal allergies, and the reference section highlighted subjects such as smoking, herbs and weight management.

Food & Fitness   go hand in hand when it comes to weight management. However, they don't seem to sit well together in this channel, which veers from features on items such as healthy fish recipes to a six-week online triathlon training programme. Better is Dr Liz Applegate's fitness nutrition page, a typical subject of which is when to eat lunch so you can still fit in a midday workout. She is an expert on nutrition and performance and an esteemed author of books on that subject. More advice from her in the archive includes 'Don't feel guilty about frozen dinners' and 'Too much of a good thing – carrot juice overload'. How refreshing...

Library   A panel at the top of this channel's homepage highlights the site's Top 5 Topics, and they are: sex, diet, symptoms, diabetes, and pregnancy. Under The Basics, you can search for information on conditions by clicking on the relevant letter of the alphabet. There is also a drug database, a vitamins and minerals guide, and a section on first aid and coping with emergencies at home or away. Under Research there is a medical dictionary and a page of recommended websites.

Community   is a key element of this site, with many of the channels relying heavily on queries from visitors to prompt editorial content and professional advice.

Toolbox   is a cut above the rest in our view, as it features a breast self-examination, Yoga at Your Desk, and a diet and fitness journal in addition to the usual calorie and nutrient calculators and body mass index calculator. The excellent medicine checker lets you cross-reference medication to avoid unwanted drug interactions, while the symptom checker evaluates your aches and pains, and the wellness manager allows you to create your personal health page. Home Delivery, which requires registration, will deliver daily or weekly emails on the type of health news you specify.

Nurse Connect   is a telephone service offered by the site in which you can consult with a registered nurse for US$9.95 per call. They will take questions on specific symptoms, women's health, infant care, children's health, men's health, and health after 60.

Links   Many, in the library section, divided into subject categories including specific conditions and general themes.

OTHER FEATURES

Shopping, USA clinic directories.

A lively site with many interesting features, particularly strong on community interaction. Unlike other sites that give you numerous reasons why they can't actually answer the questions you are supposedly invited to ask, On Health uses visitors' queries as a springboard to fine content.

www.outdoorhealth.com
Outdoor Health

Overall rating: ★ ★ ★ ★ ★			
Classification:	Information	Readability:	★ ★ ★ ★ ★
Updating:	Daily	Content:	★ ★ ★ ★
Navigation:	★ ★ ★ ★ ★	Speed:	★ ★ ★ ★ ★

US

Outdoor Health is produced by multimedia health information specialists adam.com. Although the site is dedicated to people with an enthusiasm for activities such as hiking, trekking and camping, there is a strong medical element to the information. 'Experienced explorers and backpackers alike will find the essential information they need to prepare for their next adventure,' says the homepage, which highlights the involvement of Dr Paul S Auerbach, clinical professor of surgery in the division of emergency medicine at Stanford University and author of Medicine for the Outdoors, from which most of this information comes.

On the homepage, choose from one of the topics buttons across the top of the screen or scroll down to see the highlighted features. You can search the site by keyword in the box near the top of the page.

SPECIAL FEATURES

First Aid and Emergency Care is divided into airway and breathing, circulation and consciousness, general emergencies, victim transport, first aid, procedures and pharmacological relief, so you can look up the problem and then see how to deal with it. The first aid kits section details items you need to take with you, such as topical skins preparations, wound care and splinting and sling material. There are dedicated links in the first aid kits section dealing with particular environments, such as forest, mountain and aquatic areas.

Symptoms aims to help you identify what the problem may be, whether chest pain or just heartburn, the type of diarrhoea, and so on. The section is conveniently broken up into sub-sections such as respiratory symptoms, disorientation and loss of consciousness, muscles, and bones and joints.

Major Medical Concerns 'Are you ready for an emergency?', they ask at the top of the page. The following list of categories makes it clear you're probably not, covering as it does things like treatment for severe heart attack, asthma, giving subcutaneous injections, emergency childbirth, all major fractures and dislocations, lightning strike, how to assist breathing and what to do with an unconscious victim – and that's just a brief rundown. The aim is to help you recognise and, in some cases, treat medical emergencies until the victim can be seen by a doctor. This is all the more necessary in the wilderness, where medical emergencies can be just as unexpected as in civilised areas, but more frightening to handle.

Minor Medical Concerns Minor? The first one on the list is coughing blood! But as you will discover on reading, the cause could be something as simple as a sore throat, or as disturbing as lung cancer. As we are told here, under 'What to Bring, What to Know', the key to health and safety in the outdoors is pre-trip preparation. This can be as simple as stocking up on painkillers, or as advanced as learning the proper CPR (cardiopulmonary resuscitation) technique. Instructions for it are supplied here, too, of course.

Environment-Related Concerns It's important to have an idea of potential dangers before you travel to unfamiliar environments. Here problems are listed under the climates and environments in which they might occur: illnesses and injuries due to cold, emergencies and illnesses related to high altitude, all the bites, stings, poisonings and burns that can occur in a forest, underwater dangers, plus weather-related phenomena and problems associated with natural disasters, such as what to do in an earthquake, avoiding tornadoes and lightning, and carbon monoxide poisoning. As with the other sections, all the conditions are listed alphabetically within the sections for easy reference.

Injury and Illness Prevention The best defence against sickness and injury in the wilderness is to prevent it happening in the first place. This section aims to help you do just that by outlining common-sense behaviour, trip planning, maintenance of communication, conditioning and acclimatisation tips, how to disinfect water and so on. A reference guide to immunisations is included.

Activity-Related Concerns Play hard but play safe is the message of this detailed section, divided into hiking/backpacking, running, skiing and boarding, climbing, camping, scuba diving, fishing and foreign travel. Within these categories are myriad problems you may encounter (some unique to America), which range from muscular and exposure conditions to attacks from insects, animals and reactions to plant life. Click on each link to find out about prevention, symptoms and treatment.

Q&A of the Week Click on the links at the bottom of the page to access this section, in which Dr Paul Auerbach answers questions from site visitors. The homepage of the site features a few of the questions given previously, with relevant links to other sections of the site. Typical submissions include: 'How do I safely remove a tick?', 'I want to take my 2-year-old daughter on our skiing holiday – how do I know if she is suffering from the altitude?', and 'I get blisters all the time when I go hiking – am I supposed to leave them alone or take the fluid out?' The answers given are thoroughly detailed but very easy to understand, and they include details of how to prevent problems as well as treat them.

Links To the home of adam.com, which also runs the Dr Greene parenting site.

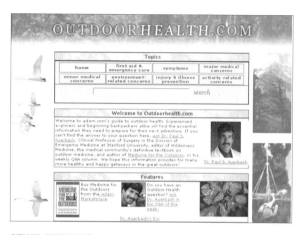

OTHER FEATURES

Medicine for the Outdoors is offered for sale.

You may not be able to log on while trekking, but Outdoor Health has a wealth of useful information that it is wise to look up before you go. As at least one reader has found, you may also want to buy a printed copy of the book to carry with you on expeditions.

www.quackwatch.com
Quackwatch

Overall rating: ★ ★ ★ ★			
Classification: Information		**Readability:**	★ ★ ★
Updating: Frequently		**Content:**	★ ★ ★ ★
Navigation: ★ ★ ★ ★		**Speed:**	★ ★ ★ ★

US

A duck kitted out in a Sherlock Holmes outfit is the logo of this highly esteemed and not-for-profit site, subtitled 'Your guide to health fraud, quackery and intelligent decisions.' The man behind it is Stephen Barrett MD, who aims to be as open as possible regarding the operation and funding of the site. It costs around $500 a year to produce, which in part explains the merely functional design and unsympathetic usability, and this money is made from the sale of books recommended on the site.

Scroll (you'll be doing a lot of it) down the homepage to read the list of channels and articles – many are ones yet to be posted, but it is useful to know that you may have a reason to come back. These include other campaigning sites that are spin-offs of key issues encountered by Barrett, such as Chirobase, the MLM (multi-level marketing) Watch and NutriWatch.

SPECIAL FEATURES

Most Recent Additions to Quackwatch, as well as the sister sites Chirobase, MLM Watch and NutriWatch, are highlighted in a page linked from under the masthead of the homepage. You can access the homepages of the sister sites from the new additions page. The anti-multi-level-marketing site may seem incongruous; however, as Barrett points out, this is how a vast number of so-called health products are sold. 'Nearly all MLM companies selling health-related products exaggerate their value.' NutriWatch, put together with the help of Manfred Kroger PhD, aims to be 'Your Guide to Sensible Nutrition', and uses the dietary pyramid as a masthead. An interesting (and quite amusing for us journalists) article was 'Confessions of a Former Women's Magazine Writer', in which the author admitted the dietary drivel she was employed to perpetuate. Here there are also dietary guidelines, nutrition basics, food safety and technology articles, topical features, and government aims.

About Quackwatch Here you'll find details of the site's mission, its legal and scientific advisers, the 52 awards given to the site since it started, other cheers and jeers, a health fraud discussion list, and a special message to cancer patients seeking alternative treatment. The latter is especially worth a look. It highlights (extensively) the way promoters of dubious treatments manipulate the emotions of desperate cancer patients and their families, and gives an overview of alternative methods with a long list of treatments named as questionable.

About Stephen Barrett MD He is a retired psychiatrist who works as a medical editor, author and consultant. He will answer questions related to consumer health by email, and the best ones are posted on the site. You are asked to search Quackwatch before sending in your question to make sure the subject has not been covered already.

General Observations Several subjects are covered here. First, quackery, with key features being '25 Ways to Spot Quackery' and 'How Quackery Sells' (there are several more along the same lines). Also here are 'some notes on the nature of science', 'why bogus therapies seem to work', and 'how to spot an internet bandit'.

Questionable Products, Services and Theories Nearly every alternative practice you can think of comes under this spotlight: acupuncture, algae products, aromatherapy,

Ayurveda, yeast allergies, Chinese medicine, homeopathy, juicing, qigong, naturopathy – that's just a few. Chiropractic comes under particular scrutiny.

Nonrecommended Sources of Health Advice targets books, advice in health food stores, organisations, nutrition consultants, websites, book publishers 'promoting' quackery, plus a long list of individuals, including some of the most famous names in alternative health: Andrew Weil (see p. 48), Deepak Chopra, Adelle Davis, Earl Mindell and Robert Atkins. Some are links to other sites rather than articles written by Quackwatch, including an extensive look at the career and thinking of Weil.

Consumer Protection includes doctor-patient communication tips, a piece on 'intelligent' consumer behaviour, antiquackery organisations, online scams, plus several other articles relating to regulations, particularly in America. Interestingly, Quackwatch is in favour of GM food production and does not believe GM foods should be labelled as such.

Consumer Strategy: Health Promotion sheds light on current popular health issues, such as the scientific perspective on antioxidants and other phytochemicals, risk factors in cardiovascular disease, tips for low-fat eating, choosing and using exercise equipment, hormone replacement therapy, vegetarianism ('healthful but not necessary'), food irradiation ('a valuable public health measure').

Consumer Strategy: Tips for Practitioner Selection includes advice on choosing a chiropractor, why you should beware of 'free foot exam', advertisements and tips on how to check a physician's credentials. Articles on choosing dentists, pharmacists, nutritionists, physicians and how to get mental help were promised as we went to press. Typical is this comment from Barrett: 'Choosing a chiropractor can be difficult because the majority of chiropractors are involved in unscientific practices.'

Consumer Strategy: Disease Management Look here if you have irritable bowel syndrome, latex allergy, lower back pain, scoliosis, glaucoma, or are intrigued by the piece on overuse of antibiotics, blood-pressure drugs and heartburn drugs. There are also tips for prudent drug use.

Education for Consumers and Health Professionals is a diverse section including critiques of recent articles and broadcasts, internet health scares, urban legends, rumours and hoaxes, evaluating websites, plus recommended magazines, newsletters and journals.

Links There are many throughout the site, plus a dedicated links section.

OTHER FEATURES

Translations into several languages, questionable advertisements, details of Quackwatch research projects, how you can help with legal and political activities.

Quackwatch is without doubt an important and useful information resource. A healthy dose of scepticism is certainly required when reviewing popular health information, especially when it encourages you to part with your money or raises hopes unfairly. However, we did find that the more we read, the more we felt it was equally important to be sceptical about the viewpoints of the sceptics, who define what is possible or true only in terms of what science has managed to 'prove' to date.

http://webmd.com
WebMD

Overall rating: ★ ★ ★ ★ ★			
Classification:	Information	**Readability:**	★ ★ ★ ★
Updating:	Daily	**Content:**	★ ★ ★ ★ ★
Navigation:	★ ★ ★ ★ ★	**Speed:**	★ ★ ★

US

A well-established site that supplies content to other major internet names, Web MD aims to be a venue for all aspects of medical health, the key site for medical insurers as well as health care professionals and patients, and very much has its eye on an electronic future of health care in the US.

On the splash page, select the consumer button at the top right of the screen to be taken through to the lively homepage, which offers a taster of the day's key news stories, as well as menu strips and pull-down menus leading to the reference sections.

SPECIAL FEATURES

WebMD Today is the catch-all name given to the news service and daily interactive 'events' flagged at the top of the homepage. Typical of the content is an article based on a recent study and related chat sessions and tips. Our last visit saw the topic 'What makes a good father?', based on the surprising results of a study, a look at the importance of father figures to kids, a chat on the 'love codes' dads use, and tips for fathers on balancing family and career. Scroll down the lengthy homepage for links to the channel's daily highlights in Hot Topics. We read about the proliferation of Prozac and US government scientists downplaying the capabilities of vitamin C to 'prevent cancer, stop heart attacks, do the dishes and wash the car'. Your Healthcare covers lifestyle issues and advice such as how to relax

through exercise and how to help adolescents deal with body image problems. Tools You Can Use are also found here, including a secure facility to organise and record your family's health care data, a target heart rate calculator and a means of appraising your general health risks.

Medical Info 'You are not alone,' says WebMD to newly diagnosed patients. You can access information on a range of conditions and diseases by selecting from the pull-down menu on the homepage. Otherwise, head to Diseases and Conditions on the left-hand menu panel, which will bring up a long list to choose from. Each ailment is presented with a few features on things such as new findings, treatment discoveries, risk factors, and so on. Links are provided to an overview, treatment and diagnosis information and to notes on clinical trials. A look under Back Pain found that some of the magnet gadgets being marketed for natural relief from aches and pains were causing potentially fatal problems for people with implanted heart devices, but that a deadly poison – a botulinum toxin – was relieving back pain when injected in tiny amounts into muscles along the spine. Where relevant, complementary therapy information is included in the reference section for each condition, so, too, self-care dos and don'ts. However, as we found with back pain, even the natural remedies such as chiropractic can have negative side effects of which potential patients first need to be aware. Prevention information is also included in some sections for those who are trying to shut the door before the horse bolts – perhaps if a problem runs in a family. Other categories within this channel are Drugs and Herbs and the Medical Library. The latter is massive and includes not only an A–Z reference guide on health topics, but also illustrated guides, a medical encyclopedia, an Ask the Experts facility, the Yale Medical Test Guide, and listings of over 35,000 clinical trials. Click on Our Content Sources to read about the authoritative sources of all this information.

Health & Wellness is like an extensive site in its own right. Living Better is just one section of it, and that alone includes ten subcategories of feature pages. We liked the Healthy Living category, which offered a choice of daily focus articles on parenting, seniors, alternative medicine, emotional wellness, and legal and insurance information. Really gutsy issues were covered, such as what to do if you have been denied surgery, whether you should stop having sugar, what to do after an adulterous affair, sibling rivalry and how to deal with a health care provider who is skimping on your prescription drugs. Also within Healthy Living is diet and nutrition information, plus sections for men and women, sexuality and pregnancy. Dean Ornish MD's Lifestyle Program is a special chapter from the American celebrity doctor and best-selling author, a champion of integrative and preventative medicine. His key point is that comprehensive lifestyle changes can reverse severe coronary heart disease and other conditions without drugs or surgery. He answers a visitor's query daily in this section, which also includes the components of his programme – nutrition, exercise, stress management, love and intimacy – and an archive of gourmet recipes that fit in with the Ornish philosophy of eating. Look under Health & Wellness, too, for a news-oriented sport and fitness section (find out how your favourite tennis star recovered from injury), and some Health-E-Tools including the typical health risk appraisal, target heart rate and body mass index calculators,calorie counters, plus less common facilities such as an ovulation calculator, kid's height predictor and pregnancy weight gain calculator.

WebMD Member Services is the wide variety of live events and interactive features offered on the site.

Links Many are included throughout the site to a variety of information and support organisations, online retailers, plus the myriad advertisers.

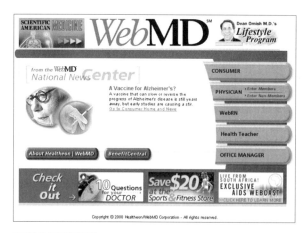

OTHER FEATURES

Health TV, About WebMD, MyHealthcare (for US audience).

Worth visiting for the Dean Ornish Program alone, WebMD is a well-organised, comprehensive and authoritative information source – a pleasure to use and certainly one to bookmark.

www.askyourpharmacist.co.uk
Ask Your Pharmacist

Overall rating: ★ ★ ★ ★			
Classification:	Homepage	Readability:	★ ★ ★ ★ ★
Updating:	Monthly	Content:	★ ★ ★ ★ ★
Navigation:	★ ★ ★ ★ ★	Speed:	★ ★ ★ ★ ★

UK

Here the National Pharmaceutical Association highlights the expert level of advice available from trained pharmacists, who can speak with authority and recognise and treat minor ailments, as well as advise on medicines and their use.

This dark green homepage has its channels arranged in a grid across the centre of the screen. As you move the cursor over each section it will light up, indicating that you can enter by clicking at that point.

SPECIAL FEATURES

About Medicines offers advice on choosing and using medicines, understanding what's on the label and how to safely store and dispose of medicines. There is also instruction on what to tell your pharmacist before you buy a product – such as who it's for, what treatment (if any) has been tried already, whether the patient has any allergies, and so on.

New This Month On our last visit, this section highlighted the special offers and giveaway competitions at chemists belonging to the National Pharmaceutical Association as part of a summer promotion to publicise the wealth of information available from your local pharmacist. Scroll down to the bottom of the page and you will find an archive of seasonally topical features, such as curing

colds and flu in winter, hay fever in spring and sun care in summer.

Directory of Pharmacies Enter your postcode or town in the search box given and the site will provide you with a list of pharmacists local to you.

Kid's Page Brad the Bear appears monthly here with a new picture and rhyme that can be printed out for colouring by children. The aim is to be educational; it is not just about how useful pharmacists are, but about the importance of taking medicine properly, not teasing children who have to take medicine at school, and so on.

Links to patient.co.uk, the BBC health news and web guide, www.winter.uk (which is an NHS site to help people choose the right remedies at winter), and the Doctor-Patient Partnership (www.doctorpatient.org.uk).

OTHER FEATURES

About Pharmacy, advertising campaigns, careers information.

'Community Pharmacy Working For You', indeed – Ask Your Pharmacist clarifies how to make the most of the professionals working in your local chemist and provides a good promotional avenue for independent chemists who do not have the advertising budgets of the big high street names. More content would be welcome, however.

www.bupa.co.uk
Bupa

Overall rating: ★ ★ ★ ★			
Classification:	Homepage	Readability:	★ ★ ★
Updating:	Daily	Content:	★ ★ ★ ★
Navigation:	★ ★ ★	Speed:	★ ★ ★ ★

UK

Bupa is one of the UK's major private health insurance providers and has designed this site as an information resource to the general public as well as a facility for its members. To access the general information, click on the Your Health button towards the top left-hand corner of the homepage. You will then be presented with an introductory page explaining what may be found in this 'healthy living' section (the information has been approved by Bupa's doctors), and offering a menu panel down the right-hand side of the screen. Alternatively, you can search the site by keyword by typing in the box at the top of the left-hand column.

SPECIAL FEATURES

A to Z Factsheets Click here and you will be offered a choice of search facilities: you can type in a keyword, or select an option from the pull-down menu. A reasonable range of conditions is offered – notably plastic surgery, which is not often covered on health medical sites. Choosing the Mental Health option brought up the opportunity to refine the search to an impressive selection of mental health problems, including recovering from drug misuse, bereavement, attention deficit hyperactivity disorder, Alzheimer's disease, alcoholism, and more. The fact sheets included general definitions and characteristics of a problem, characteristics of people at risk, typical symptoms (physical and psychological), diagrams, medical treatment, complementary therapies and outcomes of treatment.

Baby Centre This section includes the interesting results of the Birth and Motherhood survey, commissioned by Mother & Baby magazine in association with Bupa, as well as a pregnancy glossary, advice on conception from Bupa's doctors, what you need to know about the birth, and what to expect during the five months after the baby is born.

Men's Health aims to tackle the embarrassment many men feel in discussing health issues. One section here presents answers to the six nerve-wracking questions their survey reveals men would most like to ask. There are also articles on the testes, prostate, Viagra, men and cosmetic surgery, baldness and shaving rash.

Seniors' Health is not a large section, unfortunately. It offers dedicated coverage of Parkinson's and Alzheimer's disease and, like the other sections of this site, veers into cosmetic issues with tips to help you look younger than your age.

Women's Health is an interesting selection of articles, with features on cellulite, hysterectomies, period pain, infertility, breast cancer and advice on how to check your breasts.

Complementary Medicine debates the legalisation of cannabis, offers articles on popular therapies such as aromatherapy and chiropractic, plus a beginner's guide to lesser-known natural treatments, and information on herbs.

OTHER FEATURES

Latest health news, member information, About Bupa, clinic and hospital search facility, Children's Health, Lifestyle Issues, General Health Issues.

We saw the phrase 'trust Bupa' a little too often to be entirely comfortable with this site as an information resource. Some of the editorial content is very good and covers areas other sites shy away from. The company clearly has a vested interest, though this site would be very useful for current members.

www.embarrassingproblems.co.uk
Embarrassimg Problems

Overall rating: ★ ★ ★ ★			
Classification:	Homepage	**Readability:**	★ ★ ★ ★
Updating:	Daily	**Content:**	★ ★ ★ ★ ★
Navigation:	★ ★ ★ ★	**Speed:**	★ ★ ★ ★ ★

(UK)

Dr Margaret Steam – a medical doctor with an additional BA in physiology and psychology – is the expert behind this inspired site, whose slogan is 'straight talking good advice'. As the name suggests, Embarrassing Problems seeks to provide information about issues that people commonly feel too shy to ask their doctor about. It's friendly and discreet, at times humorous, but not in a ridiculing fashion. So many problems are covered it is difficult to believe there is a person on earth who would not find useful facts and tips here, and you can email the site with suggestions of topics they have yet to cover. In the two months since its launch, the most frequently visited pages have been anal itching, oral sex and wind, but you can also search here for less intimate concerns such as acne and spots, aging skin, shyness, snoring, sweaty feet, memory problems and dandruff.

There is a keyword search box at the left of the homepage. Alternatively, you can click on the button titled 'A-Z topics' and a box will leap up with a list of problems – simply scroll down it and click on the one you want to read about.

SPECIAL FEATURES

Wind Stop laughing. We all do it and, as this section reveals, most of us expel about 600ml of gas per day, although some people may produce up to 2 litres. In fact, healthy young men break wind 14–25 times a day. That's a greater volume than women generally; however, women tend to produce stronger smelling gas. Now that's something to tell your girlfriend next time she complains, and you can add this thought-provoking snippet: it is believed that trying to suppress wind can cause bowel diseases such as diverticulosis. To combat this, in the early 1990s, the Dutch National Liver and Intestine Foundation actually conducted a publicity campaign encouraging people to break wind at least 15 times a day. It's not just beans and fizzy drinks that produce gas in the bowel, either. There are an astonishing number of causes, including chewing gum or pen lids, wearing tight pants, aging, feeling stressed and bearing children. Once information such as this has helped you to feel better about your condition or situation, tips are given to help minimize the problem, and to disguise it.

Doc Spot is a monthly feature from Dr Steam, with an archive of previous subjects. Sometimes one of the conditions is featured, with questions asked by 'Blushing Bob' (a cartoon chap with a bag on his head), and on other occasions she may expand on recent headline news, such as why sweaty armpits in men can be subliminally sexy. Dr Steam has also written on finding health information on the net, how to talk to your doctor, and visiting a genitourinary clinic.

Links to Pharmacy2U and Think Natural (see p. 122 and 128), and sites with recommended products (such as www.flatulence-fileter.com).

OTHER FEATURES

Many and varied other conditions, book sales, privacy policy.

A fascinating site to surf, even if you don't have a problem or feel particularly embarrassed.

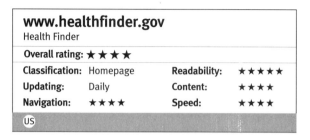

www.healthfinder.gov
Health Finder

Overall rating: ★ ★ ★ ★

Classification:	Homepage	**Readability:**	★ ★ ★ ★ ★
Updating:	Daily	**Content:**	★ ★ ★ ★
Navigation:	★ ★ ★ ★	**Speed:**	★ ★ ★ ★

US

The US government – more specifically its Department of Health and Human Services – was so concerned about the level of untrustworthy health information on the internet that it decided to build its own gateway site, linking the general public to credible sources. The homepage is easy to navigate, with a keyword search box at the top of the screen and the various channels of information listed below.

SPECIAL FEATURES

Hot Topics Look here for the Top 20 search topics each month (in fact, 26 are given). AIDS, alternative medicine, cancer, diabetes, food safety and tobacco seem to head the list. Also here: depression, pregnancy and child care, Alzheimer's disease, domestic violence, nutrition, physical activity and more. Click on a subject and you will be presented with two lists: one of web resources, one of organisations, with a link to more specific details about the resource including the URL, sponsoring agency and a description of the content.

News changes daily, drawing primarily from government, professional and web news media. Information on the latest research comes from the National Institutes of Health or the Centers for Disease Control and Prevention. When you click on this button, you will be presented with a choice of links to 'the latest', then government health news and the rest. Our last visit saw Health Finder covering the latest 'proof' that an apple a day certainly could keep the doctor away because of its high antioxidant content, as well as the development of a promising new tuberculosis drug.

Smart Choices The idea here is that the US Department of Health and Human Sciences has hand-picked documents and organisations that will help you make better, more informed health choices. Prevention and self-care (including nutrition, physical activity, oral health and mental health), first aid, support groups, doctors, health care and insurance are covered, though not all documents, especially the latter, are relevant to non-American visitors. There are also some risk assessment analyzers.

More Tools lists online libraries, medical journals and dictionaries, databases, health site search engines and foreign language resources, plus some facilities such as toll-free health information numbers that are relevant only to Americans.

Just For You specifies links for various age groups, men and women and special populations. A look under 'professionals' revealed a section specially for those in the health industry rather than lifestyle advice for yuppies. This is a good way of surveying the various parts of the site that may be particularly relevant to you. For example, the women's page revealed that hot topics for females are breast cancer, depression and domestic violence, that amongst the 'Smart Choices' channel we should take particular note of the frequently asked questions page of the National Women's Health Information Center, plus pages on preventing birth defects and the incidence of AIDS in women. We were also pointed to recommended communities for working mothers, divorced women and retired women.

Provided you are prepared to sift out the material relevant only to American residents, this is a useful resource for keeping up to date with credible health news and research.

www.patient.co.uk
Patient UK

Overall rating: ★ ★ ★ ★			
Classification:	Directory	Readability:	★ ★ ★ ★
Updating:	Daily	Content:	★ ★ ★ ★ ★
Navigation:	★ ★ ★ ★	Speed:	★ ★ ★

UK

Two medical practitioners, Drs Beverley and Tim Kenny, from Newcastle-upon-Tyne, edit and maintain Patient UK 'with the intention to direct non-medical people in the UK to information about health-related issues'. They are well known in the field of patient information, and have produced a database of Patient Information Leaflets (widely used by GPs as a supplement to consultations) for many years. Here, British sites are the primary links, but there are some links to selected overseas sites. The homepage is very easy to navigate – simply choose a subject button from the list down the left-hand side of the screen.

SPECIAL FEATURES

Medical and Health News is highlighted on the homepage and divided into UK headlines, International Health News and a page for other health news sites. Content is derived from major publications and bureaux such as the New York Times, Mayo Clinic Health Oasis (see p. 16), Ananova (the Press Association), Financial Times and the BBC. Some of it is of interest to the general public, but there is also much here that would appeal only to professionals or those with a very serious interest in the subject.

Health Related Events are updated weekly and are typically based on charity activities and promotion campaigns. Our last visit saw the Ride for Health being highlighted, along with National Osteoporosis Month and Male Cancer Awareness Month. There is a link to Future Events from the Health Education Authority diary.

Links Disease/Illness, Stay Healthy, Child Health, Women's Health, Men's Health, Seniors' Health, Eye Health, Dental Health and Travel Health are the main buttons offered on the homepage, although further down on the left is a facility for searching Scoot, to find contact details of various health and medical facilities and services in your local area. Once you click on a subject button you will be taken through to a search page for that subject, which gives you the option of searching by keyword, or by letter of the alphabet, which is handy if you have a specific condition you want to look up and don't know how to spell it. You will then be presented with links to a variety of sites on the web, with a brief outline of what they are and where they come from. Typical sources are Health in Focus (see p. 14), Medinfo, Royal College of General Practitioners and specific support groups, such as the Arthritis Research Campaign. Scroll down the page for non-UK sites and medicine information databases.

More Options is a pull-down menu that presents a variety of further site classifications, including hospices, charities, phone advice, benefits, carers, ethical, private health, medical journals and more. Beneath it is a button for links to self-help and support groups.

Add Sites You can't just add a site – which is good. You can, however, submit a site to Patient UK for inclusion. It will be reviewed by a GP to decide its suitability.

Glossaries features links to UK and non-UK medical dictionaries. Scroll down the list for glossaries that are disease- or condition-specific, such as the AIDS Glossary, Brain Tumour Patient's Dictionary, Diabetes Dictionary, and so on.

If you have a specific condition you want to find out more about, a quick search here could cut your surfing time substantially.

www.planetmedica.co.uk
Planet Medica

Overall rating: ★ ★ ★			
Classification: Information		**Readability:**	★ ★ ★ ★ ★
Updating: Daily		**Content:**	★ ★ ★ ★
Navigation: ★ ★ ★ ★ ★		**Speed:**	★ ★ ★ ★

UK

Dr Rosemary Leonard is a key contributor to this site, which also features medical professionals such as Dr Yvon Gall and registered nurse Hilary Ward-Hartley. It is put together by a 'leading pan-European eHealth company' with sister sites in countries such as France, Germany and Spain. More are scheduled for launch in the coming months, including one based in Canada. Some of the articles are clearly written by contributors in other countries and feature interviews with doctors and other specialists from there. They are, however, usually translated to an acceptable standard.

The company's practical experience is highly apparent in the straightforward and 'undesigned' layout of the site. It's refreshing to visit a homepage of such clarity – you immediately know where you are and where you could go, and are tempted to explore by the highlighted features with good photographs listed down the centre of the screen. Planet Medica's tone is that of a serious women's magazine, and articles putting a timely and informative spin on bras, skincare and parenting are typical of the content.

SPECIAL FEATURES

Top 5 seems to be the subjects searched most frequently. On our last visit these were managing stress, couples' sexuality, antidepressants, breast cancer and migraine. Click on each of these and you will be taken through to a magazine-style feature from elsewhere on the site, such as

Ten Ways to De-Stress at Your Desk, or Sexual Harmony is Achieved by Listening, with links to other features at the bottom of the screen or in a box to the right. Alternatively, you may be given a list of reference topics you can then choose from.

Your Wellbeing is a large section comprising 'news, views and expert advice on how to look after yourself and feel your best everyday'. In practical terms, this means sections dedicated to fitness and relaxation, diet and weight, nutrition, sexuality, pregnancy and birth, plus alternative medicines. We found the poorly-translated piece on Diet Cooking very disappointing and not up to Planet Medica's usual standard. Better were the ideas for shaping up without going to the gym: how to tone pecs and buttocks while commuting, or sit at a desk and lift heavy objects correctly.

Medical Conditions offers an alphabetical search facility of ailments plus quick links to the most popular subject areas: breast and prostate cancer, anorexia, osteoporosis, fibroids, alcoholism, back pain, and so on. Clicking on anxiety took us through to a brief definition of the condition, and offered a lengthy feature article by Dr Danny Allen on how to deal with someone who is always anxious. There were also links to an anxiety test, related features on mental illness and psychotherapy, similar conditions like panic attacks and schizophrenia, and a dossier entitled 'what do we know about anxiety?'

Test Yourself offers a two-minute psychological profile 'to find out what kind of person you really are!' There is also a series of symptoms assessments for various conditions. Click here and you will be presented with a list of topics including 'Are you addicted to tobacco?', 'Do you feel sleepy during the day?', 'Eating Attitudes Test', 'Sexual Arousability Inventory', and so on.

Medicines Planet Medica acknowledges that this index of medicines is not exhaustive. However, it is their aim to make it so. You can search for information alphabetically or choose a medicine family or class from the lengthy pull-down menu. Choosing antidepressants from the latter took us through to a page explaining types rather than brands available, a round-up of how they work, plus links to pages on mental health conditions, depression, anxiety and depressive states. There are also links in this channel to news about medicines and drugs.

Doctors and Hospitals is potentially where the British sites score over the otherwise well-produced American ones. However, all this section does is offer the facility to search for types of healthcare professional, hospitals, clinics and surgeries through Scoot. You could have gone to Scoot for that. The promise is that 'this is where to locate the right healthcare facilities for you', but it's not that personalised. Nor could we find the advertised pieces on how to prepare for a hospital appointment and communicate with medical professionals – maybe they will be there by the time you read this.

Communities offers a newsletter for 'all the latest health news from Planet Medica', as well as message boards. At the time of our last review these were not particularly well attended or lively.

Medical Library contains several sections, including news from Reuters, special reports from medical experts, an archive of stories from Your Wellbeing, results of the Planet Medica polls, and an A–Z medical encyclopedia. Choose news and you will be presented with a chronological list of stories. Content veers from new drug launches and scientific discoveries to EU activities and new medical reports. The Quick Votes reveals that only a slight majority of site visitors disapprove of animal testing, most would not have cosmetic surgery in the light of recent health scares, and 80 per cent want more realistic body shapes in fashion magazines and television ads. There is a lot of good information in the Medical Encyclopedia, which veers into lifestyle subjects

such as achieving proper nutrition and personality development for teenagers, but not all of it is brilliantly translated.

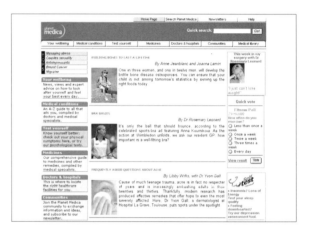

All the basics are here to make a top-notch site, but Planet Medica needs more consistency in the quality of its editorial content for British consumers. Its appeal is that it is less commercial and flashy than sites such as NetDoctor.co.uk.

http://surgerydoor.co.uk
Surgery Door

Overall rating: ★ ★ ★ ★			
Classification:	Information	Readability:	★ ★ ★ ★
Updating:	Daily	Content:	★ ★ ★ ★ ★
Navigation:	★ ★ ★	Speed:	★ ★ ★

UK

Surgery Door claims to be Britain's most comprehensive health website and features Dr Mark Porter, celebrity medico, as its lynchpin contributor. Instructions for navigating the site, which operates by frames, are supplied as part of the welcome on the homepage, which also has links to the weather, TV listings and daily news. The day's selection of features is listed down the centre of the page, with health news headlines scrolling across the top like a tannoy. You can search the site by keyword using the box at the top left of the screen.

SPECIAL FEATURES

Health Daily The inclusion of a weather forecast on this site doesn't seem so ridiculous when you consider the benefit to hayfever sufferers of knowing the pollen count, or to asthma sufferers of hearing about areas of high air pollution, and the increasing importance in our lives of UV rays. These are included in the Health Daily channel along with a health events diary, news, a daily selection of tips on a chosen health subject (such as treating bruises and sprains), and monthly pages from Dr Mark Porter, which include answers to posted queries. Also here is a link to the Radio Times listings of television and radio programmes and the Sunday Mirror newspaper.

Medical Emergencies, the first section of this channel, is highlighted in yellow on the menu panel and provides brief advice on how to recognise emergency medical situations

and what to do in them. It includes a paragraph describing the recovery position, a step-by-step guide to mouth-to-mouth breathing, and what to do in cases of chest pain and shock. Look to the right of the screen for links to types of emergency: bites and stings, animal bites, broken limbs, injured neck and spine, and the like. Other channel content includes an index of signs and symptoms (types of bleeding, breathlessness, and so on), a first aid primer, and what to include in a home medicines chest. Outside the emergency section is a guide to prescription drugs, a medical dictionary, a self-medication guide, support group listings, and more. A section on organ donation discusses the major transplant procedures and the National Organ Donor Register, and gives both case studies of successful operations and Dr Porter's view on the subject.

Healthy Living Preventing accidents, dental health, drugs, alcohol, smoking, healthy eating, vitamins, sexual health, new parents, health and beauty – this channel is nearly as large and diverse as the Medical section. Advice in the sports health and fitness section comes from Lilleshall National Sports Centre, and here you can find tips on choosing a gym as well as all the components of a good workout programme. In Good Health, Good Sex (which 'go together like bees and honey or beans on toast', we are told) there is advice on how to recharge your sex life, herbal remedies and what to do when you suffer loss of libido, plus a directory of sexual dysfunction in men and women, and answers to the question 'Is this normal?' from agony aunt Julia Cole. Look in Healthy Homes for advice on combating the 30,000 deaths annually in the UK due to winter-related illnesses such as avoiding condensation, and energy conservation tips.

NHS & Benefits Your NHS is intended as a guide to help people understand more fully the National Health Service today and obtain the services they need, but it is rather confusing to use. First click on the alphabetical list to narrow your search – under A you will be presented with categories such as 'Access', 'Adolescence', 'Alarm Systems', 'Ambulance Services', and 'Appointments'. The information is all approved by the NHS. Health in Your Area is a listing of doctors, dentists, opticians, and so on throughout the UK, and can be searched by typing in your postcode and selecting a service from the pull-down menu. You will be provided with contact details and a map to the facility. Benefits and Entitlements includes leaflets to download from the Benefits Agency plus a brief explanation of the circumstances under which a person may be entitled to benefits – there is a long list of situations to peruse including maternity leave, sick pay, child benefit, employment rehabilitation allowance, and so on.

Complementary Medicine features an A–Z of therapies, plus an introduction to the most popular treatments, including chiropractic, acupuncture, homeopathy and osteopathy. Selected support groups are listed below them. Did You Know highlights the finding that nearly two out of every five general medical practices offered some form of complementary medicine for NHS patients and discusses the gap between complementary and conventional medicine.

Travel Health covers vaccinations needed in a country-by-country guide and suggests a list of items to include in a traveller's health kit.

Community & Fun includes message boards, quizzes and competitions, 'patient experiences' of various conditions and ailments (you can email in your story), a health survey and similar interactive facilities.

Shopping The Surgery Door Multistore claims to have over 20,000 products including medicines and toiletries, beauty products, disability and lifestyle aids, natural bodycare, aromatherapy, organic foods, vitamins and minerals, books, videos and magazines, and even flowers and chocolates (are they to take to patients you know?). These are all links to established internet retailers such as Pharmacy 2 U,

ThinkNatural.com, Thorntons, Interflora, and so on. There is a special offers section.

Links to retailing sites, support networks, government organisations, and so on, with a special links page from Dr Porter and a 'Research Your Health' link to the US National Library of Medicine.

There is a tremendous amount of good and useful information here, but it could be much better organised and designed. This weakness may be due in part to the site simply having so much content. In trying to be all things to all people it includes several peripheral subjects that seem like clutter – no good when you're trying to find information quickly (Surgery Door could learn a few things from Web MD). But persevere and you will probably discover much you did not know about health and the health service in the UK.

OTHER SITES OF INTEREST

Organising Medical Networked Information and Biome
http://omni.ac.uk and http://biome.ac.uk
As we went to press, these sites were joining forces and planning a massive relaunch. Omni has been a key gateway to medical information services for around five years and, teamed with Biome, will expand to include all health and life sciences: agriculture, food, pharmaceutical sciences, medicine, nursing, dentistry, biological research, veterinary sciences as well as forestry, botany, zoology and more.

British Medical Association
http://web.bma.org.uk
The prestigious British Medical Association often makes the news here and internationally, whether through raising awareness of health and medical issues, reports in its British Medical Journal, comments on the state of the industry, or its responses to external events and moves by government. Aimed primarily at the medical industry, with official comment and press releases, it is interesting for those with a serious or professional interest.

Nursing Standard Online
www.nursing-standard.co.uk
Nursing Standard is the premier magazine for the nursing industry, but this site is more a homepage for the magazine than an information resource. It offers insight into nursing campaigns and issues, news headlines and files for downloading. In a similar vein, emergency-nurse.com aims to provide an online focal point for emergency nurses, rather than advice on what to do in a crisis.

Department of Health
www.doh.gov.uk
The British government's Department of Health website is intended for use by health and social care professionals, academics and interested parties. There are links to other health-related sites, plus press releases that may be of interest to the general public – typical subjects are the government's research reports, comment from ministers, and pledges of support or attention to various issues.

The Quality Information Checklist
www.quick.org.uk
Produced in part by the Health Education authority, this is a cartoon-based guide and tool for teachers, which also contains tips relevant to us all when it comes to assessing the quality of health information we are presented with on the net. It explains clearly and simply what questions to ask yourself about a site, and why.

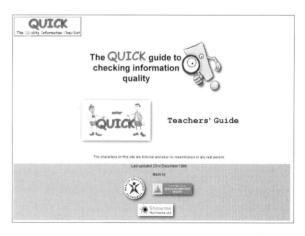

The Online Medical Dictionary
www.graylab.ac.uk/omd
Sponsored by BT and compiled by Dr Graham Dark, this site contains over 65,000 terms relating to many aspects of medicine and science, and includes acronyms, jargon, theory, standards, institutions, projects, – 'anything to do with medicine or science'. It's easy to use: simply type in the word you are looking for and press the search button. You can also view the contents by subject area or starting letter.

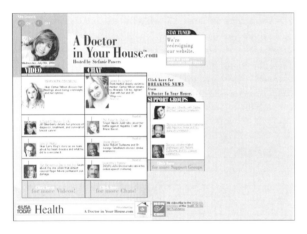

Health on the Net Foundation
www.hon.ch
A Swiss organisation, Health on the Net Foundation – or HON – is a not-for-profit group that aims to improve the quality of healthcare information on the net, and make searching for it easier. To this end they have several projects on the go, including an industry code of conduct and a programme of research into usage of the internet for healthcare purposes, and you will see their distinctive logo on many sites you visit using this book. This site also offers health information to individuals, and you can, for example, visit its support communities for information on aging, allergies, hepatitis, vision and eye care. The library contains papers from conferences and other medical sources.

Health Gate
www.bewell.com
American medical and healthy living sites are myriad – click on the 'About Us' buttons and they're all talking about e-solutions and investment opportunities and, for the most part, they're all pretty much the same. This one allows its writers longer articles than most. We couldn't find any celebs amongst the contributors, but enjoyed the content.

A Doctor in Your House
www.adoctorinyourhouse.com
If OK! magazine were a health website, this would be it. A Doctor in Your House is hosted by Hart to Hart actress Stephanie Powers and concentrates on American actors, singers, chat show hosts, and so on who have faced and conquered health problems. It's not as bad as it sounds. Carnie Wilson of Wilson Phillips (and the daughter of Beach Boy Brian Wilson) has her own obesity support community as well as video footage of her laparoscopic gastric bypass surgery on this website. Also here, Maurice White of Earth Wind and Fire discusses neurological challenge, Larry King tells of his experiences with heart disease, and Roger Moore reveals his brush with skin cancer. Go on...admit you want to read it.

United States National Library of Medicine
www.nlm.nih.gov
The United States National Library of Medicine (NLM) is an information source and gateway to other medical sites on the web, and is most beneficial to professionals and anyone undertaking intensive research into a subject. Some of the content applies only to the American market. You will find

a complete list of the NLM's searchable databases and databanks, details of research programmes and clinical trials. Interesting facets are the History of Medicine Division and the Visible Human Project, which creates anatomical images of the male and female human bodies.

InteliHealth
www.intelihealth.com
You don't need to visit InteliHealth to read its material – it is distributed to many high-traffic sites, including America Online, DiscoveryHealth.com, women's site Lifetime Online, and the prestigious Washington Post newspaper. The site claims to be 'the trusted source' and aims to 'consumerize' health information to make it accessible to the widest possible audience. The site is well done, divided into channels for women, men, children, seniors, with daily news, lifestyle articles, analyzers, and so on – all the typical stuff on other general medical sites is reviewed here. Which you prefer is simply a matter of personal preferences regarding tone and ease of use.

Consumer Health Information Centre
www.chic.org.uk
The Consumer Health Information Centre has been specially set up to advise the general public on health matters. At this site you will find reliable and entertainingly presented health information on topics including men's health, cold and flu, de-stressing, pain and what to put in a home medicine chest.

British Dental Association
www.bda-dentistry.org.uk/public/
This link takes you directly to the public pages of Britain's leading association of dental practitioners. Here you will find a very good set of frequently asked questions about dental care, files of treatments to download, list of recommended toothpastes, toothbrushes, mouthrinses and floss, and a search facility for dentists in your area.

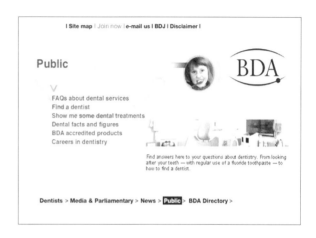

Dr Koop
www.drkoop.com
Dr C Everett Koop is a former US Surgeon General, one of America's most charismatic celebrity doctors, but also renowned for his down-to-earth approach. His eponymous site incorporates conventional medicine as well as lifestyle issues, self-care advice and alternative medicine, and is worth checking regularly for the amusing column, 'A Word from Dr Koop'.

Chapter 2

complementary medicine

A recent British Medical Association (BMA) report on acupuncture revealed that nearly half of the doctors surveyed would like to receive training in acupuncture in order to treat their own patients in future. Now, that would be 'integrative medicine', wouldn't it?

While cautious about the lack of Western-style clinical research into acupuncture's effectiveness, the report acknowledged that evidence suggests acupuncture is more effective than 'control interventions' for back pain, nausea and vomiting, migraine, and dental pain. Best of all, the study found that 79 per cent of GPs would like to see acupuncture provided on the NHS (it's now available in around 86 per cent of NHS chronic pain services), and called

for further research into its effectiveness, plus the establishment of a single regulatory body of practitioners.

It's been a long time coming – hundreds of years – for Western medicine to acknowledge formally the benefits of even well known complementary therapies such as acupuncture. Surely it is only a short mental leap to recognise that if acupuncture is effective, acupressure and shiatsu, which work on a similar basis but without needles, could offer some relief too?

In the past practitioners of such therapies have suffered from a hippy-dippy image, but public dissatisfaction with the state of hospitals and unpleasant drug side effects means an increasing number of 'normal' people are prepared to consider the benefits of complementary therapies and seek out treatment.

Nevertheless, that's all the more reason to be careful. The boom in the complementary therapy and alternative medicine in the last few years has led to a dramatic increase in practitioners and, indeed, new therapies being developed, some of which are really quite left of field. It's essential to take charge of your own health by becoming as well-versed as possible in your condition and the therapies that may benefit it. That's where the internet can help. The sites recommended here can tell you what a healing method is, what it can and can't do for you, how to find a good practitioner and what to expect when you go for your appointment. It is certainly worth taking a look at www.altmedicine.com in which health journalist Frank Granzian makes a point of focusing on 'proven' information, and for balance cross refer with www.quackwatch.com (see p. 28), the ultimate site for sceptics.

www.altmedicine.com

Alternative Health News Online

Overall rating: ★ ★ ★ ★

Classification:	Gateway	Readability:	★ ★ ★ ★ ★
Updating:	Daily	Content:	★ ★ ★ ★
Navigation:	★ ★ ★ ★	Speed:	★ ★ ★ ★ ★

US

This multi-award-winning site was founded by journalist/publisher Frank Granzian with the aim of providing visitors with credible alternative health and wellness information. Hundreds of links are given to key alternative health sites such as Ask Dr Weil (see p. 48), plus favoured traditional medicine sites, including the British Medical Journal and The Lancet. The homepage explains the goals and points to bear in mind while reading this and all other health information, whether on the internet or not, and you are encouraged to read it. Enter the site at the bottom of the page, and you will be presented with a large menu.

SPECIAL FEATURES

What's New is updated daily to help you save time when searching for the latest health news. The page is simply huge, with probably every major health news story listed and introduced in a few sentences for time-effective browsing, which is a much better approach than sites that provide only the opening words. You then click on the link to find out more. You will be taken to the site of the story but without leaving Alternative Health News Online, and can use the back button to return to the list of articles. The aim is to report the news objectively, so many controversial studies are included, some of which may not agree with establishment views.

Health News Bulletins differs slightly from the What's New section in that, rather than reporting all the news, it aims to notify visitors of the major research findings and developments based on scientific reports and statements from authorities – stuff that is considered proven rather than simply a theory. This has been a key part of Granzian's mission: to let people know what is proven and separate the genuine from the junk. Some of the stories are cross-referenced to other relevant articles. Again, the list of entries is massive.

Search Engine Wow, this is good! You can search the site by keyword, or click through the link to another five top medical search engines containing millions of entries. We tested a few conditions on the site's search engine. Usually, a great many articles were presented. Equally interestingly, on the occasion when only one entry was given, it was a fascinating report that we had not found on any other site when searching the same subject.

Diet & Nutrition, like most of the other categories, contains a carefully considered list of recommended links, plus some diet and nutrition tips, which are accompanied by short articles explaining the principle. You will discover a lot of good stuff here not found elsewhere.

Mind/Body Control Not just yoga and hypnosis, but humour therapy, prayer therapy, music therapy, art therapy, biofeedback and a choice of meditation styles. Amongst the Mind/Body Tips section was news that people who have challenge, commitment and control in their jobs are less likely to be stressed and that cutting stress may prevent cancer, and some proven methods of relaxation and de-stressing.

Alternative Medical Systems are the ancient systems of healing that have served non-Western cultures perfectly well for thousands of years and are, today, increasingly seen as alternative options rather than weird practices. Here are links to key pages on homeopathic, naturopathic, Chinese, Ayurvedic, environmental and holistic medicine.

Manual Healing primarily involves the hands, and there are pages on chiropractic, the Feldenkrais method, Trager method, rolfing, cranial osteopathy, therapeutic touch, massage, reiki, qigong, reflexology, osteopathy, Alexander technique and aromatherapy. Amongst the tips was advice on preventing stress injuries such as carpal tunnel syndrome by performing simple exercises when working at the computer, news that water pillows seem to be better for chronic neck pain than other pillows, and proof that acupuncture aids stroke patients.

Longevity is for the elderly and those who would like to stay young. Look here to find advice on eating to stay young, how to age healthily, guides to health and exercise for seniors, the site of the Ageing Research Centre, and more. Things you can do now to help increase longevity include eating fruit and soybeans.

Books We Recommend is not about book sales to fund the site, it's books they really do recommend. Subjects range from non-diet diets to mindfulness, an alternative medicine ratings guide, and one on how to be mentally and physically active in old age.

Health News is a link to www.all-natural.com (see p. 58), which itself offers a choice of links to daily news sites covering medicine and health, such as USA Today, CNN, the New York Times, ABD News, Reuters and Healthfinder, the gateway consumer health information site from the US government.

Bookmarking this site is a must for those interested in alternative treatments and new health research, even if it is essentially a collection of links. We love the objective journalistic perspective, the way it is organised for time-effective browsing, the breadth of coverage, and the principle of distinguishing between proven facts and theories.

Dr Andrew Weil is one of the world's leading practitioners of complementary and integrative medicine; he's a fully qualified medical doctor as well as a specialist in alternative therapy, and has become quite a celebrity.

Designers of this diverse magazine-style site have carefully built it to appeal to unconfident web users, and there is a special section for first-time visitors, as well as a help section with a site map. Navigate using the panels on either side of the screen or click on one of the highlighted features.

SPECIAL FEATURES

The Best Diet in the World offers dietary and recipe suggestions based on particular ailments. There are several to choose from in a section titled Food as Medicine. The recipes here are from the doctor himself, and far more delicious than most diet food.

Q&A It's not called Ask Dr Weil for nothing. He answers a daily question from site visitors, and in this section you will find the day's subject plus a library of previous responses. The Top Ten Questions highlights the most popular queries each month. Topics extend from the benefits of vitamin C and cooking a low-fat barbecue to the psychological advantages of nudism and how to buy running shoes. We love the thoughtfully written, detailed answers.

Self-help includes the healthy lifestyle programme from Dr Weil's book, *Eight Weeks to Optimum Health,* in interactive form (really, really excellent even if it is repurposed content) and a guide to herbal medicines. The Vitamin Adviser takes the form of a quiz, with interesting notes supplied as you answer each question. At the end you receive a personalised supplement programme.

Interact With Us includes the first-time users guide and frequently asked questions, plus message boards so you can communicate with other site visitors. A free bulletin is also offered. Weekly Inspirations is a bulletin on relaxation techniques, spirituality, and healing.

In the Kitchen is written by Alice Waters, a legendary American chef admired for her expert cooking of seasonal produce, and ethical philosophy of food production. Vegetable lovers, gardeners, and foodies will love this section. Alice answers questions from site visitors in wonderful detail and offers delicious recipes.

OTHER FEATURES

Daily poll, Farmer's Market Finder (US), newsletters, book and vitamin sales.

Dr Weil has surprised many in the health industry by having a site sponsored by a vitamin company – they expected such an esteemed figure to maintain strict independence – and fans of his books may find the lack of controversial opinion on this chatty magazine-style site a disappointment. However, for those new to his style of integrative medicine and preventative health care, this is an excellent starting point, and the cross-reference linking of information between the various sections is superb.

www.wholehealthmd.com
Whole Health MD

Overall rating: ★ ★ ★ ★ ★

Classification:	Information	Readability:	★ ★ ★ ★ ★
Updating:	Daily	Reliability:	★ ★ ★ ★ ★
Navigation:	★ ★ ★ ★ ★	Speed:	★ ★ ★ ★

US

Anyone frustrated with conventional medicine, and sick of hearing from their doctor that integrative medicine is a load of mumbo jumbo, should take a look at this American site from a large group of medical doctors with training and experience in alternative fields. American WholeHealth Inc is the US's fastest-growing provider of integrative medicine, with centres in Chicago, Washington DC, Denver, and Boston. They publish this site in conjunction with a top New York-based health publishing company.

The homepage is clearly arranged with the channels listed down the centre right of the screen. As you move your cursor over each link, brief details will appear at the left offering a taster of what can be found in that channel. Alternatively, you can search the site by keyword using the box at the very top right of the screen.

SPECIAL FEATURES

Healing Centers 'Rather than prescribing powerful antibiotics or surgery to treat chronic conditions, we prefer to combine the best of conventional medicine with alternative therapies to help the body strengthen and then heal itself.' This channel is billed as the beginning of your 'healing path'. Use the alphabetical listing of conditions to start your research. You will then be taken through to a lively page offering an overview of the subject from a doctor at the centre, links to details on the courses of supplements they recommend, plus news on the latest discoveries, treatments and controversies regarding the condition. The overviews include self-care tips, an analysis of current medical treatments and advice on the circumstances in which you should call a doctor for face-to-face consultation. You can jump to these particular sections of information using the menu panel at the right of the screen, and also find out more about the doctor's qualifications to advise on the subject by clicking on the biography link beneath their picture.

Healing Kitchen offers wholefood recipes, healthy makeovers of traditional favourites plus articles on nutrition. Our most recent visit included an explanation of why tomato ketchup could be considered a health food (it contains lycopene), but to be wary of claims from product manufacturers because of the large amount that would have to be eaten to gain significant benefits.

We admired a trio of interesting potato salad recipes that were attractively illustrated and accompanied by an article on potato varieties. The rejigged version of a reader's favourite unhealthy recipe of cheese enchiladas included an explanation of how the new dish was developed, and proved a good source of healthy cooking advice that you could then apply in your own kitchen; a nutritional breakdown was provided, too.

Cool Stuff talks about new products on the market and explains why they are good in culinary and nutritional terms. Clicking on Food Remedies will take you through to an alphabetical list of conditions. Choose one in order to receive a roundup of what you should eat and why, arranged by vitamin/mineral with a list of good food sources below .There is also a satisfying list of 'mega-recipes' specially devised by the kitchen staff to contain at least 25 percent of the recommended daily intakes of nutrients for that condition. Recommended for chronic fatigue syndrome were tempting dishes such as fettuccine with mussels and spinach, roast salmon with lentils and lemon and coriander dressing, pasta with sardines and fennel, Asian crab cakes, and pumpkin cheesecake with an oat and walnut crust.

Ask Our Experts features a timely question of the day plus coverage of recent questions. On our last visit people wanted to know whether eating local honey could help relieve symptoms of hay fever, if yoga was effective for migraines or Chinese healing foods helpful for fibromyalgia, what can be done for irritable bowel syndrome when you seem to have tried everything, and whether or not a newborn baby girl's diet should be supplemented with vitamin D to help prevent osteoporosis. Amongst the speciality fields of the experts featured here are Ayurveda, Chinese medicine, chiropractic, herbal therapies, homeopathy, mind-body medicine, nutritional therapy, and women's health. Click on the menu panel to the right of the screen to browse the archive.

Reference Library is divided into therapies (from acupuncture to yoga), supplements (acidophilus to zinc) and foods (almonds to yogurt), plus safety and usage information for more than 750 drugs and 'the essentials of wholehealth', which includes nutritional basics, supplement use and safety, and choosing the best multivitamins. You will also find an exclusion diet for allergy sufferers here.

News and Perspectives typically includes a timely feature story, media and product reviews, plus news stories from around the world. Our last visit, in summer, saw tips on using essential oils to keep bugs at bay while on picnics, research from Norway revealing that exercising four or five times a week cuts the risk of a stroke in half, a move from British researchers to print the minutes of life lost through smoking on each pack of cigarettes, and a review of a book entitled The Yoga of Herbs, put together by Ayurvedic practitioners.

My WholeHealth requires site registration and allows you to save articles and recipes from the site to a personal file that will help you access information particular to your health more quickly and easily.

OTHER FEATURES

Shopping, find a practitioner (US).

An informative, comprehensive, and professionally run site that could easily inspire you to play a positive role in your own health management.

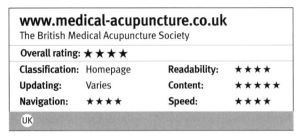

www.medical-acupuncture.co.uk
The British Medical Acupuncture Society

Overall rating: ★ ★ ★ ★

Classification:	Homepage	Readability:	★ ★ ★ ★
Updating:	Varies	Content:	★ ★ ★ ★ ★
Navigation:	★ ★ ★ ★	Speed:	★ ★ ★ ★

UK

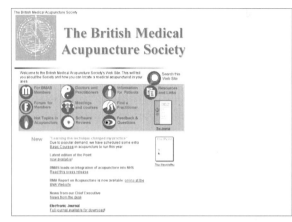

The British Medical Acupuncture Society is a group of family doctors and hospital specialists who practice acupuncture alongside conventional Western medical techniques. The aim of this site is to help UK residents find a medical acupuncturist in their area. However, some information is provided for consumers and professionals.

Beneath the main menu panel in the centre of the screen there is a list of new additions to the site. You can also search the site by keyword – just click on the search icon.

SPECIAL FEATURES

Hot Topics in Acupuncture is a selection of serious articles on the subject, including the use of acupuncture in NHS general practice, current scientific understanding of the practice, and an explanation of the differences between medical and non-medical acupuncturists.

Information for Patients A key concern of this group is the unsubstantiated claims made for acupuncture, because they tend to confuse rather than enlighten. This section explains the practice of responsible acupuncture and its uses, plus its past, present, and future, and gives general information on how to find a practitioner. An interesting fact is given under Where to Go for Acupuncture: 'At the moment, anyone in the UK is allowed to call themselves a doctor and start advertising and practising acupuncture

immediately, regardless of qualifications and experience.'

Find a Practitioner Some of the society's members are given under this link, which features areas in the UK that you can then click on for a list of local practitioners.

OTHER FEATURES

On the site are links to the Society's Journal and its newsletter, The Point (ha ha). Outside links are to a variety of acupuncture research articles, international acupuncture societies, publications, diagrams, case studies, news-groups, and much more. There is also a forum, plus information and resources for members.

This site must be your starting point when looking for a responsible acupuncturist in the UK.

www.healingpeople.com
Healing People

Overall rating: ★ ★ ★ ★			
Classification: Infomation		**Readability:**	★ ★ ★ ★
Updating: Varies		**Content:**	★ ★ ★ ★
Navigation: ★ ★ ★ ★ ★		**Speed:**	★ ★ ★ ★

US

Healing People is a multi-faceted site that aims to be a key source of reference for complementary and alternative medicine information. Many of the staff are alternative therapy practitioners and the site boasts an advisory board of more than 40 other experts.

Although the design is attractive, it is not a good site for small screens. You will have to make the window as wide as possible and still may have to scroll horizontally to read the right of the page. The main types of therapy are listed down the centre of the screen; at the left are various resources, while current features are highlighted to the right. There is a keyword search facility beneath the logo at the top of the screen.

SPECIAL FEATURES

Chinese Medicine   This section was formerly called www.acupuncture.com, but it includes other forms of Chinese healing that don't require needles! You will find information on Chinese nutrition, TuiNa and acupressure, t'ai chi and qigong, herbology, plus testimonials from satisfied patients and resources for professionals and students. Amongst these are anatomical drawings featuring all the acupuncture meridians. These practices have been serving the Chinese well for around 5000 years now, making one wonder about just how 'alternative' they really are. The information, however, would be better served with

a more consistent structure and writing style. Sometimes the articles are little more than a series of one-word bullet points.

Homeopathy   The subsection titled An Introduction to Homeopathy includes several articles, ranging from how homeopathy works and its place in alternative medicine to homeopathy from your garden, the ten most common homeopathic medicines, homeopathy for babies, and why psychotherapy and homeopathy are 'the perfect marriage'. Also here is a series of articles on conditions treated by homeopathy, such as asthma, coughs, diarrhoea, migraine, hyperactivity, and insommnia.

Western Herbalism incorporates the use of vitamins, minerals, and plant extracts in the prevention and cure of illness and is considered particularly good for depression, anxiety, menopausal women, PMS, asthma, indigestion, colds and flu, as well as other problems. As articles in the introduction to the subject explain, typical remedies are St John's Wort, echinacea, Siberian ginseng, and other products widely available in health stores, chemists, and supermarkets. The Herbs section of this channel offers a series of articles on these specific herbs – good old garlic is featured, too.

Nutrition & Lifestyle includes two main subsections, titled Exercise & Lifestyle and Food & Nutrition. Included amongst the former is a 'total life stress quiz', an article on Ayurvedic fitness or yoga, a chakra flow meditation, and advice on tension headaches. Food & Nutrition is a much larger section, with articles on a diverse range of subjects, including specific health reports, vegetarianism, drinking milk, the role of magnesium in depression, macrobiotics, nutrition for allergies, and a great deal more.

Ayurveda   There's more yoga here, plus segments on Ayurvedic herbs, conditions treatable by the practice (colds and flu, attention deficit disorder, candidiasis, migraine, constipation, some cancers and obesity, amongst others) and a general introduction to the subject including its history, how Ayurveda works, and the most frequently asked questions.

Aromatherapy is perhaps the most pleasant of all alternative therapy treatments, involving as it does being lightly massaged with beautiful smelling oils. This section provides a guide to the oils used and, for anyone doubting its effectiveness, a series of articles on some of the more serious medical conditions aromatherapy can offer relief from, including nail fungus, irritable bowel syndrome, headaches, Alzheimer's disease, infections, and hair loss.

Bodywork is a small section that covers frequently asked questions about massage and other hands-on practices, plus some cautions and contraindications to be aware of.

Cancer Risk Reduction Healing People claims to be on a mission to promote awareness about the avoidable risks associated with cancer. This section highlights the foods, cosmetics, household and garden products said to be carcinogenic and aims to promote safer alternatives for everyday use. Articles include 'We are losing the winnable war against cancer', 'Facts on carcinogens at home', and the thought-provoking 'Perfume: Cupid's Arrow or Poison Dart?'.

Pet Health Homeopathy for dogs, chiropractic for cats, flower remedies for your horse... it's all here, along with veterinary acupuncture.

More How could there be more? Well, there is, and here you'll find vibrational medicine, energy medicine, allopathic medicine, cranial electrical stimulation, naturopathy and, believe it or not, healing poetry. But we had to laugh when we saw that they forgot humour therapy.

General Encyclopedia aims to give the most up-to-date, research-based information on disease, symptoms, treatment, remedies, and supplements. You can search alphabetically by subject category. The entries are lengthy and detailed, with all the research references listed at the bottom.

Healing Communities Users are required to register before participating in the various noticeboards offered. Some are for healthcare professionals, others for patients, discussing alternative medicine in general and specific treatments.

Ask Healing People offers the opportunity to post questions to the site's resident practitioners of homeopathy, Ayurveda, and acupuncture, and find out if their treatments could benefit you.

OTHER FEATURES

Online Store, Suggestion Box, Professional Encyclopedia, Practitioner Listings, FAQ, Newsletter, and links to a variety of natural health sites and articles.

While this site has been put together with the best of intentions, and is backed by an impressive list of professional advisors, we felt that as a publishing venture it was inconsistent and not well structured. There is a lot of interesting and unique information to be found here, but it is not presented in a way that is most useful to the reader: some of the articles are technical and in-depth, and others are mere lists with little explanation, rather like a student's lecture notes.

www.internethealthlibrary.com
Internet Health Library

Overall rating: ★ ★ ★ ★

Classification:	Ezine	Readability:	★ ★ ★ ★ ★
Updating:	Daily	Content:	★ ★ ★ ★ ★
Navigation:	★ ★ ★ ★	Speed:	★ ★ ★

UK

The Internet Health Library is the 'official health information provider' of the British Complementary Medicine Association. It offers the general public a range of articles and fact sheets about alternative therapies and is careful to emphasise that the material is unbiased and free – apart from the homeopathic consultations, for which there is a charge. They also want to make clear that the information provided is fully referenced and, interestingly, the site refuses to acknowledge animal-based research on the basis that results of animal testing cannot be extrapolated to the human species. As the editors point out, aspirin kills cats, while sheep can swallow enormous quantities of arsenic.

The homepage, while lively, is a bit of a mish-mash. There are navigational strips across the top and down the left-hand side of the screen, with special offers, competitions, and some features highlighted at the centre of the page. There is a site search facility at the top left-hand corner of the screen. It's difficult to know where to start.

SPECIAL FEATURES

Main Index should probably be one of your first ports of call: trying to browse the site without having read it could lead to confusion about what is where. It lists the key sections of the site and briefly outlines what can be found in them.

Health Problems A-Z can, as the title suggests, be searched alphabetically. Click on the ailment or condition you want to read about and you could be presented with a fact sheet on causes of it, or perhaps with reports of research into useful alternative treatments for a problem.

Alternative and Complementary Therapies also works as an A–Z and covers more than 50 practices, from the well-known acupuncture, massage, and naturopathy to less common Australian Flower Essences therapy, bee venom therapy, marma therapy, music therapy, and chelation therapy, plus exercise, yoga, and tai chi. The entries are not always detailed.

Products and Services is an alphabetical list of treatments that have been registered with the Internet Health Library. When we clicked on Ayurveda we were taken through to an advertorial-style article on a health spa. It sounded good for a holiday sometime, but a list of local practitioners would have been more useful.

Diet and Nutrition is the first entry in the box titled Health Matters. Click here and you will be presented with a list of vitamins and minerals, which is not in itself helpful because it works on the theory that you already know what you need. However, choose iron, for example, and you will be presented with an informative fact sheet detailing what it is, factors that influence its absorption, its function and signs of deficiency, plus a list of related links down the right of the screen to recommended daily intakes, best sources, articles on anaemia, and Ayurvedic medicines.

Diet and Lifestyle offers a diverse list of articles and papers for reading including food combining, the Dead Sea, complementary therapy dentistry, health benefits of dealcoholised red wine, longevity, macrobiotics, prayer, sports medicine, the herbal first aid kit, and much more. Sources include the American Journal of Clinical Nutrition, Acupuncture in Medicine and other professional magazines, university papers, and so on. The information is good, but pulling together such disparate subjects under this general chapter title is unhelpful and you may be better off searching the site by keywords.

Surveys concentrates mainly on research findings regarding attitudes to complementary therapies, such as a Which? survey showing public support for alternative medicines, a professional publication's statement that 40 per cent of GPs in the UK are now referring patients to complementary therapists, and a Mintel report revealing that sales of dietary supplements continue to rise.

Environmental Health Clicking here opens a new window that will take you through to pages from the environmental organisation Friends of the Earth – or rather, it does some of the time. There seemed to be several bugs in the system on our last visit.

Women's Health offers a list of conditions and other topics peculiar to the female of the species, including anorexia nervosa, cervical cancer, various subjects related to pregnancy and childbirth, endometriosis, and premenstrual syndrome. You will then be presented with fact sheets and useful links to organisations and related articles.

Children's Health runs in a similar way to Women's Health, but the fact sheets are helpfully categorised into general subject areas such as breastfeeding, vaccination, children's health problems, and so on.

Online Homeopathic Clinic This service is available for a selected number of common ailments. It stumbles at the first hurdle, from a user's point of view, in that we have to diagnose ourselves. Do irritated nasal passages and a sore throat suggest the onset of a cold or sinusitis? There's nothing in this section to tell you, and no links provided to symptom checklists. Then there is the poor wording on the questionnaire: PMS sufferers are supposed to tick a particular box if they have swelling in the abdomen and particularly sore breasts. What if you get one but not the other? Do you tick or not? If you suffer from painful periods but not anaemia, are you supposed to tick the box that lumps them together? If you fail to type in your county in the address box (who on earth specifies a county after London?), the site registers an error and wipes the whole form so you have to fill it out again. Other than that, we rather like it. It's only £14.95, and treatments are sent out first class within 24 hours.

Links to support groups, Friends of the Earth and other authoritative sources of information, professional associations, training colleges, as well as advertised services.

OTHER FEATURES

Health headlines, what's on, press releases, courses, suggestion box.

This site suffers from poor organisation of the material, but what's here is good, authoritative, and easy to read.

www.windsandwaters.com
Winds and Waters Chinese Healing

Overall rating: ★ ★ ★ ★			
Classification: Ecommerce		**Readability:**	★ ★ ★ ★ ★
Updating: None		**Content:**	★ ★ ★ ★
Navigation: ★ ★ ★		**Speed:**	★ ★ ★ ★

CAN

Although this easy-to-navigate and cleanly designed site operates as an online retailer, it offers a wealth of fine introductory information on traditional Chinese medicine (often called TCM). From the homepage, click on TCM Theory to access the explanatory articles.

SPECIAL FEATURES

TCM Theory compares and contrasts traditional Chinese medicine with Western medical practice, arguing that the conventional Western medicine concept of a cure cannot be applied successfully to the increasing number of viruses as they do not respond well to antibiotics, and anti-viral drugs can have bad side effects. People under the care of TCM practitioners are expected to take an active role in their health by changing unhealthy habits. Interesting stuff, and this section breaks down into the following components:

Concepts Most of us have heard of Yin and Yang. Here they are explained.

Pathogens explains why we get sick, and is divided into environmental, mental, and other factors such as eating, personal behaviour, and stagnation.

Organs explains briefly the Chinese theory of how organs work.

Organ Function describes each organ and their symptoms of illness. These are divided into Zang and Fu organs, plus the brain and uterus. Chinese and English names are provided for the key words and concepts.

Diet Yin and Yang food is covered in this brief section. Its purpose is to encapsulate the basic theories, such as raw food is more cooling than cooked food; plants that take longer to grow such as cabbage, carrots and parsnips are considered Yang in nature; chewing food thoroughly creates Yang warmth, and so on.

TCM Practice explains what you are likely to experience in a consultation with a Chinese medicine practitioner, including methods of evaluation and diagnosis, questions you may be asked, what they will be looking for when examining your tongue, face, and body language, taking your pulse, and sniffing you.

Using and Preparing Herbs explains how to make the traditional Chinese herbal soups that are inevitably prescribed.

This is an excellent introduction to Chinese Medicine, clear in words and design. However, it is important to note that online diagnosis is not a reasonable alternative to face-to-face consultation. A practitioner of Chinese medicine cannot look at your tongue, take your pulse or sniff you via email from Canada.

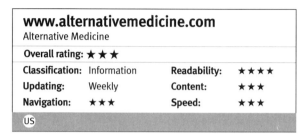

www.alternativemedicine.com
Alternative Medicine

Overall rating: ★ ★ ★			
Classification:	Information	Readability:	★ ★ ★ ★
Updating:	Weekly	Content:	★ ★ ★
Navigation:	★ ★ ★	Speed:	★ ★ ★

US

The homepage of this site, which claims to be 'the internet's largest database of alternative medical information on how to get and stay well', is quite off-putting, as it appears to be sales rather than information-oriented. That may be because the publisher, Burton Goldberg, is a businessman, which is in itself rather unusual in the alternative medicine field. He says, 'Our website, books and magazines... represent the collective wisdom of thousands of alternative physicians and practitioners worldwide who are practising the medicine of the future today for your benefit.' Be patient – there is some really fascinating stuff here.

SPECIAL FEATURES

What's Hot is a weekly article (previous features are archived) on a timely issue. At the beginning of summer it may be treating ear infections to coincide with an increase in swimming; at the beginning of the new year it focused on weight loss. The articles are long and detailed, and a little difficult to read with all the biological and technical names.

Search Health Conditions   A keyword search can present you with several articles from various sections of the site in response to your query. We were highly impressed by some of the tips given in the articles, which incorporated treatments as diverse as nutritional therapy, herbal medicines, biofeedback light stimulation, aromatherapy, and acupuncture on our searches. There's a wry sense of

humour at work here too, with one feature headlined 'Depression is not a Prozac deficiency' and others looking at dietary supplementation and acupuncture as a means of mending a broken heart. Most entries are written by alternative health practitioners and other experts, whose details are given at the bottom of each piece.

Political Issues are topical essays on selected subjects. As we went to press the need to label genetically engineered food was being highlighted – a subject that is only seriously being discussed in America now as a result of British campaigning on the subject.

Provocative Essays are written by Burton Goldberg, and they cover subjects such as the cost of health care, longevity, alternative medicine, the difference between 'scientific' and 'proven', cancer treatment, and resisting the prescription of antibiotics.

OTHER FEATURES

Yellow Pages (US), clinic listings, message boards, book, magazine and product sales, opinion poll, newsletter, and more.

There is some excellent information here and very handy advice on health conditions. It's just a pity it's arranged and designed so badly.

www.all-natural.com
Natural Health and Longevity Resource Center

Overall rating: ★ ★ ★

Classification:	Homepage	Readability:	★ ★ ★
Updating:	Weekly	Content:	★ ★ ★ ★
Navigation:	★ ★ ★ ★	Speed:	★ ★ ★

US

The aim of this site is to keep visitors up to date with the latest discoveries and healing methods from round the world. The site is basic in design and very easy to navigate. On the homepage, click on one of the buttons at the top of the screen to access your chosen section, or scroll down for the Nutritional Influences or Health Nutrient Profiles. Clicking on each button opens a new window, so close it to go back to the main menu.

SPECIAL FEATURES

Article Index is divided into Health Enhancement, Health Hazards, and Mind and Spirit. The list of topics is extremely long and some are links that will take you away from the site. All the typical subjects are covered here, plus some unusual ones such as the healing traditions of Noni in the Tahitian Islands, magnetic therapy, Gulf War syndrome, the true nature of reality, and how to get good results when you pray.

Health News is recommended by www.altmedicine.com. Here there are links to the major daily health news service on the net and below that is a list of links (with a round-up) to specific stories of interest to site visitors.

Guide to Nutrients is an alphabetical listing of nutritional remedies and what they can do for you. It runs from acidophilus and apple cider vinegar down to watermelon seeds, whey and zinc via all the main vitamins, minerals and herbs, plus cruciferous vegetables (broccoli etc). The latter still don't receive much publicity as cancer-fighting agents, probably because it's difficult for someone to tizzy them up and sell them at a ridiculous premium.

Guide to Herbs Not just herbs here, but flowers and roots, some fruits, and sea vegetables. Some explanations are a short sentence, others somewhat longer, but basically this is a simple reference guide.

OTHER FEATURES

Very many links, as the site predominately links to health and medical sites, but there is also a separate links page. There are also natural health products and books for sale, Health Watch, and a subject index.

A basic natural health guide that may prove an interesting gateway to new research and theories. It goes just a little further than the natural health information provided on many of the large, commercial, magazine-style sites and is well respected in the natural health community.

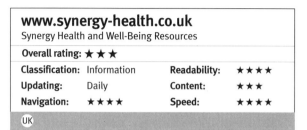

www.synergy-health.co.uk
Synergy Health and Well-Being Resources

Overall rating: ★ ★ ★			
Classification:	Information	Readability:	★ ★ ★ ★
Updating:	Daily	Content:	★ ★ ★
Navigation:	★ ★ ★ ★	Speed:	★ ★ ★ ★

UK

Based in Glasgow, this UK site has the tone and style of an enthusiasts' page. It aims to put visitors in contact with therapists and information that may be useful to them. The homepage presents a menu panel at the centre of the page, with links to the various sections.

SPECIAL FEATURES

Health and Nutrition includes health news, links to articles, testimonies about specific supplements, a list of organic food distributors, and recommended books that are for sale through Amazon.

Medical offers the opportunity to search the Rx Prescription Drug Database, which gives information on drugs that don't work together, details of side effects, and contraindications.

Diet is a brief introduction to the Hay Diet, with a table of compatible and incompatible foods. This is hardly the be all and end all of diet in relation to natural health – and the Hay Diet is a highly controversial method even amongst practitioners, not because it is dangerous but because many believe the theories on which it is based to be untrue. Still, many people feel better eating this way....

Therapists includes a directory of therapists in the UK, which can be searched by selecting the therapy and region you are interested in from the pull-down menus. A very wide range of therapies is listed, although we were surprised to find that there were no practitioners of several popular therapies listed for the Greater London area. Therapists can click on a link to join this directory. Also here is a list of professional organisations for various conditions, treatments, and practices.

What's New? has particular products for sale, such as Tahitian Noni juice, a trendy remedy everyone seems to be talking about, and Crystal Energy Water, available by mail order through Synergy.

OTHER FEATURES

A large range of links is divided into health, spirituality, neural-linguistic programming (NLP), link partners, and a Top 25. Some of these are to the informative homepages of particular practitioners. There's also an event diary, free listings, and societies.

The site really needs more participation from therapists before it can be a truly reliable information source for consumers, but it covers a lot of therapies not well known in the UK and so may be able to put you in touch with the right person. As a venue for those interested in alternative health, it doesn't have as much content to offer as the leading American sites.

OTHER SITES OF INTEREST

Deepak Chopra
www.chopra.com
Deepak Chopra has been described as the 'poet laureate' of alternative medicine but he tends to work more in the field of spirituality and philosophy than medicine, alternative or otherwise, especially in books such as To Know God and The Seven Spiritual Laws of Success. 'It is the mission of our organization to heal, to love, to transform and to serve,' he tells us on this site, which is really just a homepage for his activities, courses, and workshops in the US. It's not to be confused with www.deepakchopra.com, which claims to be the world's largest discussion forum for his fans and offers to send you an inspirational message each day 'to help you progress on your spiritual journey faster'.

The Ayurvedic Institute Info Center
www.ayurveda.com/info/index.html
This address takes you straight to the articles section of the Ayurvedic Institute based in New Mexico. It's mission is 'to promote the science and art of Ayurvedic medicine and the betterment of public health via Ayurveda', which is considered by many to be the world's oldest healing science. Choose the article you want to read from the pull-down menu. There is an introduction to Ayurveda by Dr Vasant Lad, an author of many books on the subject, who achieved his Masters of Ayurvedic Science in India and has practised for many years in the USA. He has also written a piece on incompatible food combinations according to Ayurveda. Sadly, the pages are not easy to read.

Feldenkrais Guild of North America
www.feldenkrais.com
Feldenkrais is a method that aims to teach the body a functional awareness of the self in the environment. 'What?', you say. Basically, it's a way of improving your well-being by using the body fully. However, it is not, as this site explains, a medical, massage, bodywork or therapeutic technique.

Why bother? It is said to be beneficial for those experiencing chronic or acute pain in the back, neck, legs, and so on, as well as those who suffer from problems of the central nervous system such as stroke, multiple sclerosis, and cerebral palsy. Many seniors also enjoy using the technique as a means of helping them move freely. Anyway, you can find an in-depth explanation of it here.

Biorhythm Chart
www.facade.com
Hey boys, would you like to see Cindy Crawford's biorhythm? Well, you can here, although there's little point in knowing it. Type your own birth details over hers, however, and the site will calculate your anticipated physical, emotional, and intellectual states for a given day or set period. The theory is that our lives are affected by these three primary cycles and, when they are at a high point, it is easier and more beneficial to do things that require aspects of that trait. It's not a form of divination, however. This site will also assess your 'secondary' biorhythms, which are cycles of passion, wisdom, and mastery, and see how they compare with those of your significant other, or, indeed, Cindy Crawford.

National Federation of Spiritual Healers
www.nfsh.org.uk
'It's gentle, it's natural and it works,' says this British group of practising spiritual healers, a registered charity founded in 1955. The healing involves the channelling of energies by the healer to re-energise the patient to deal with illness and injury. Here you can read the group's definition of the practice, look through some frequently asked questions, locate a healer near you, and find out more about what the federation does.

Shiatsu in London
www.users.globalnet.co.uk/~shiatsu
London-based practitioner Nick Clark has produced a good introductory guide to shiatsu, a gentle Oriental bodywork

practice often found to benefit sufferers of PMS, depression, chronic stress, migraine, circulatory problems, irritable bowel syndrome, and many other conditions. It is also a pleasant treatment one can enjoy as an alternative to massage and, unlike most forms of massage, the client remains fully clothed during the session. This site explains why you might want to arrange a treatment, what to expect during the session, and how shiatsu can help relieve stress in particular. In addition to providing contact details for Clark himself, it gives links to several other practitioners.

Acupuncture Self-Help Clinic
www.acupuncture-clinic.co.uk
Although this is the initially uninviting site of an acupuncture clinic in Harrogate, Yorkshire, it contains very good pages on acupressure techniques you can easily perform on yourself to relieve various problems. Choose the Acupressure Self-Help button at the right of the homepage to be taken to simple general instructions on performing the technique and a list of buttons categorising various ailments: joint and muscular pain, digestive complaints, period problems, and so on. Choosing the relevant one of these will take you through to a brilliant diagram and instructions for applying pressure. There is also a section on ear acupressure arranged in similar fashion.

Chinese Healing
www.chinesehealing.com
Are you too yin or too yang? Do this simple quiz and use the results to adjust your diet for enhanced well-being. Also here is a collection of simple recipes that, according to traditional Chinese medicine, treat common ailments.

Natural Healing UK
www.natural-healing.co.uk
This is a bit of a waste of a good domain name, since it offers visitors very little in the way of information. However, there is a search facility for British natural healing practitioners that may prove useful. You simply type in the style of treatment you are looking for (aromatherapy, shiatsu, and son on) and the site will present a list of practitioners around the UK and their contact details.

Randall Sexton's Asian Bodywork Homepage
www.asianbodywork.com
'The purpose of this enthusiast's site is to promote Asian Bodywork as one of the three great branches of Asian medicine,' says Randall Sexton. Amongst the articles are titles such as 'Zen Shiatsu for the Jet Age' (which covers overuse of computers as well as jet lag), 'Zen and the Art of Breast Maintenance', and 'Shiatsu for ME: a Positive Push'. The latter is taken from Proof magazine and features the inspiring stories of several people who feel that their ME has been relieved by shiatsu.

Dr Edward Bach Centre
www.bachcentre.com
Dr Edward Bach's flower remedies, produced in Oxfordshire, have achieved an international reputation as a gentle form of healing, particularly in relation to moods. This is the regularly updated website of the centre that was his home, and it remains the key source of production and information on his flower remedies. 'In everything we do we aim to maintain the simplicity and purity of Dr Bach's work, in the way he intended,' they state.

Chapter 3

healthy living

It's best, of course, not to get sick, and even the most conventional of Western doctors agree that the lifestyle choices we make on a daily basis have a significant impact on our state of health. Smoking is, as we all know, a bad habit and one that doctors are increasingly insisting patients must give up before true healing work can begin.

But insisting on constant perfection does no one any favours, and the mindset it perpetuates can also be damaging. According to Joanna Hall (www.health-e-lifestyle-co.com), one of Britain's leading lifestyle consultants, it's not what you do today in itself that makes a difference, but what you do today and tomorrow and the next. 'Be consistent,' she advises. 'It does not have to be 100 per cent of the time – aim for 80 percent and you are a winner.'

The sites featured here can help you shift the balance of health in your favour. They are about living well and being good to yourself (rather than being good) on a day-to-day basis. The internet is a marvellous source of inspiration, whether it be easy, enjoyable tips for prolonging life or advice on living in the moment – and actually the latter helps you do the former. So visit these sites regularly: you may even find that some of them soon take the place of your favourite printed magazine, many of whom have wisely established a presence online.

Humungous is the only word to describe this network of 700-plus sites that aims to make searching the internet easier by editing your favourite subject for you. Even the subdivisions within the Health and Fitness section show what a broad church the subject is, with categories on everything from fitness and wellness to death and dying. About.com's problem is that the larger and more successful it has become, the more complex and exhausting (rather than exhaustive) it has become too. The medical section is produced in association with Onhealth.com (see p. 24), but our focus here is on the healthy living parts of the site. On the Health and Fitness splash page, scroll down to fitness/wellness for a list of sub-categories, each a site in its own right.

SPECIAL FEATURES

Exercise is hosted by the multi-talented Jason Daniel Henderson, a certified personal trainer, former professional basketball player, web developer, and actor/model. He covers several interesting subjects, from aerobics to exercising at work, and building fitness with a disability. There is a forum within this section that veers inevitably into weight loss and nutrition – you can check it out without registering by clicking on Guest Access.

Low-Fat Cooking is a diverse section covering most aspects of cookery. It has recipes and articles on specialist cooking equipment such as bread machines and crockpots, plus features on specific ingredients such as tofu, pasta, and beef. Salt-free cooking is also covered, and tools such as meal-planners are offered to help you plan a sensible food intake.

Nutrition is an excellent, up-to-the-minute site hosted by Rick Hall, a trained dietitian and member of America's key nutrition-related organisations. It's not just about healthy eating and dieting but covers the whole spectrum of nutrition, including nutritional therapy, food safety, science, and education. The latest research is always discussed and linked to related features and subjects, and while Rick is not afraid to tackle controversial subjects (for example, anti-soy research or suggestions that lactose intolerance can be decreased by drinking more milk), he aims to take a balanced, long-term view. It's a pleasure to visit for serious nutrition-heads who want to keep well-informed.

Running/Jogging gives plenty of advice for beginners on training programmes and clothes, as well as a vision of how extreme their chosen sport could become: there are sections devoted to ultrarunning and running psychology, and the site makes it clear that it's not so much about winning races or losing weight as Zen and the meaning of life.

Walking Britain is only just beginning to take walking seriously as a means of fitness – in America and Australia it's big news, so reading these pages can fill walkers with a sense of longing rather than satisfaction. For example, in the US there is a phenomenal range of shoes available for walkers, but not in the UK, where we are typically expected to wear running shoes or, indeed, to take up running. Beginners will find advice on how to walk for fitness, what to wear, how to cope with injury, treadmills, or hot weather, and for the serious enthusiast there's advice on how to prepare for races, marathons, and ultrathons, where you could walk across an entire country or continent. Trekking is covered too, along with walking holidays and worldwide walking events, and if you need any more inspiration, there are articles on famous walkers.

Weight Loss It certainly can't be said that this site takes a dictatorial approach to weight loss advice: it's unafraid to cover controversial trends and fads like low-carb eating, the Dr Atkins diet, cabbage soup diet, or the blood-type diet. It's enough to make a state-registered dietitian weep. There are sections here too on body image, children's weight issues, diet pills, fasting, medical methods of weight loss, eating disorders, a link to the exercise section covered above, and forums for visitors to swap tips and ideas. In covering so many theories and dubious claims, the site may actually prove confusing rather than helpful, and while there is a section on weight loss for teenagers, we reckon only responsible adults should be surfing here. The heading for the fad diets section encapsulates their position: 'Fad or just unorthodox?'

OTHER FEATURES

Other subjects covered include bicycling, bodybuilding, martial arts, senior health, sexuality, spas, swimming, tennis, and vegetarian cuisine. Each section has its own community features such as message boards, and a comprehensive selection of links annotated by the site host.

A comprehensive resource that does not hesitate to tackle awkward or way-out subjects, but visitors need to maintain a level head, particularly when reading the community-based sections and pages on extreme diets. We want to stress, even before our lawyers force us to, that advice offered by members of the general public is never a substitute for consultation with a doctor or health professional.

www.bbc.co.uk/health
BBC Health and Fitness

Overall rating: ★ ★ ★ ★ ★			
Classification:	TV Webpage	**Readability:**	★ ★ ★
Updating:	Daily	**Content:**	★ ★ ★ ★
Navigation:	★ ★ ★ ★	**Speed:**	★ ★ ★ ★

UK

This BBC site has a broad remit, covering health issues from serious news headlines to soap plots. The homepage is packed with entry options including highlighted features in the centre and menu strips along the top and down the left. Even more is to be found in the pull-down menu headed 'Health sites listed by category', and there is a box for searching the site by keyword at the top right of the screen. Flash is required for some sections and Mac users are advised to browse using Netscape Navigator rather than Internet Explorer. This is disappointing – a site of this provenance should be designed to be easily accessible to all surfers.

SPECIAL FEATURES

Men's Health is divided into four main sections addressing body, mind, lifestyle, and life-span, featuring a pertinent 'countdown calculator' designed to prompt chaps to look after their health. There are tips on recognising and coping with stress and depression.

Women's Health is, perhaps amusingly, rather more girly than the men's health section and includes beauty pages on acne, cellulite, and cosmetic surgery. However, there's also more comprehensive coverage of mental health issues such as post-traumatic stress, obsessive-compulsive disorder (men don't get these?), and of course a section on reproductive health. Your Body includes general information on fitness plus pages on osteoporosis, menopause, eating disorders, and exercise addiction.

Kid's Health is a fun, how - things - work section for children, rather than advice for parents (which is covered in parenting). This section includes a tour of the body and addresses mental health by encouraging children to talk about what's worrying them.

Parenting is produced in association with the Health Education Authority and includes advice for parents-to-be as well as those coping with newborns and toddlers. Common childhood illnesses and immunisation are addressed too.

Travel Health makes going on holiday sound incredibly dangerous – you could get frostbite or sunburn, get bitten by bugs or snakes, get diarrhoea, drink dodgy water, have an accident, go to a dangerous area, or encounter drugs, alcohol, or people you might want to have sex with. After scaring you off going anywhere at all, they offer a section called Prepare and Prevent which advises on jabs, what to take, and how to prepare your mind by eliminating expectations that everything will be perfect.

Health in Soaps EastEnders, Doctors, Holby City, and Casualty are nothing like real life – or are they? This section might seem silly but in fact the last decade has seen many popular soaps covering health and medical issues in a responsible fashion, not only tackling difficult subjects but offering telephone support lines and information sheets to address viewers' concerns and answer questions raised.

Kick the Habit contains plenty of archived material for people interested in giving up smoking. Although the campaign had recently finished at the time of writing, and some information is not strictly current, there is much to support people in their desire to give up smoking, for example Dale's Diaries, in which popular presenter Dale Winton chronicles his efforts to give up cigarettes.

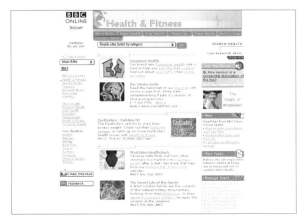

Fighting Fit, Fighting Fat is another old campaign archived for reference, and – judging by attendance on the message boards – one of the most popular, which continues to generate much interest. It's intriguing that so many people ask questions of other dieters when they would perhaps be better off seeking the advice of a professional. Nevertheless, the main section includes many sound recommendations on eating well, being active, assessing your body mass index and maintaining enthusiasm for your weight-loss project.

Ask the Doctor features a daily question answered by professional GPs, and an archive of previous questions categorised alphabetically. The responses are detailed and helpful.

Your Guide to... Here there are several sites within the site. The large section on ageing is very well put together, lively, informative, credible but fun – the BBC at its best. There's also coverage of subjects such as hormones, back pain, allergies, and arthritis.

Webguide is a weekly selection of health and fitness sites to visit. This is very well organised and gives a brief explanation of each site's purpose and content rather than merely the name and link. There's an archived list of previously featured webguides.

OTHER FEATURES

News, quiz, vote, weekly newsletter, related programmes, and links throughout the site to support and information organisations.

Informative, responsible, excellent in almost all respects, this is much more than its classification of TV homepage might suggest, and is not restricted to regurgitating or promoting telly programmes. If this is where the licence fee is going, we're happy to pay it.

www.clickmango.com
ClickMango

Overall rating: ★ ★ ★ ★			
Classification:	Ezine	Readability:	★ ★ ★ ★ ★
Updating:	Fortnightly	Content:	★ ★ ★ ★ ★
Navigation:	★ ★ ★ ★	Speed:	★ ★ ★ ★

UK

'Click into nature' and 'A mango a day' are the slogans of this natural health and beauty site that aims to help people help themselves to a better life. The co-founders are two blokes who seem to be rather evasive about their past, but editorial director Catherine Baudrand and consultant Sally Pearce bring credibility to the outfit, having been leading figures on women's magazines before joining the company. Page layout encourages visitors to click on one of the featured articles to begin surfing and offers many entry points. The top right-hand blob contains a menu of the main sections, which are Wisdom, Shopping, and Community.

SPECIAL FEATURES

Wisdom is a reference section encouraging you to 'Learn, Discover, and Heal'. Choose from Health, Nutrition and Diet, Glow, and Natural Therapies from the menu strip at the top of the page, or click on one of the highlighted features. Advice and tips come from industry experts such as holistic beauty therapist Bharti Vyas, natural health practitioner Michael van Stratten, The Times medical columnist Dr Thomas Stuttaford, holistic vet Richard Allport, and aromatherapist Lotte Rose. Recipes and other food information are taken from van Stratten's previously published books, while skin-care info is from Vyas's book *Beauty Wisdom*.

Community includes some celebrity features plus advice from the previously mentioned experts. You can post questions to them, but unfortunately they answer very few, which rather defeats the object. The limited number that are addressed are answered in depth, but it's quite possible to read through the featured questions and find nothing of interest. The message boards redress the balance a little as many of the discussion topics are initiated by the experts. The Chat section advertises online chats with them and invites visitors to book a place. Joanna Lumley's Absolutely Natural column focuses on alternative treatments tried out by her, and Celebrity Health interviews women in the public eye about their natural health habits and how they keep in top form.

Shopping ClickMango has an exciting range of products for sale, including several brands that you may have read about in magazines but not been able to find locally, such as Liz Earle, Yin Yang, Nonie of Beverly Hills, Dessert Essence, and the Bharti Vyas range. Search by condition, lifestage or brand from the pull-down menu on the homepage, or click on a type of product from the menu panel beneath. Food includes special teas, organic fruit and nuts, sports supplements, and baby food. There are Chinese herbs and tinctures too. For an overview, click on What's New, where chief buyer Janaki Nicholas chooses her monthly favourites.

Newsletter Every fortnight, site host Joanna Lumley, in full Ab Fab mode, introduces new additions to the site and suggests why they may be of interest.

Encyclopedia of Family Health This is an online version of a book previously published by Hamlyn. Each week a selection of different conditions is highlighted, such as indigestion, stress, or PMS.

Although this site incorporates a lot of previously published material, the editorial is interesting, and the shopping's Ab Fab.

www.feelgooduk.co.uk
Feel Good UK

Overall rating: ★ ★ ★ ★			
Classification:	Ezine	Readability:	★ ★ ★ ★ ★
Updating:	Daily	Content:	★ ★ ★ ★ ★
Navigation:	★ ★ ★ ★ ★	Speed:	★ ★ ★ ★ ★

UK

Part of the iCircle network of women's sites, Feel Good UK nevertheless offers good medical and fitness information for men and children as well as women. Natural health is covered by its iCircle colleague Think Natural (see p. 128). The menu panel on the homepage highlights several categories such as breast cancer, contraception, migraine, pregnancy, stopping smoking, a gynaecological clinic, and infertility. Topical features are highlighted at the centre of the screen, and may include a response to a health issue highlighted by celebrity news such as Patsy Kensit's struggles with panic attacks, or a seasonal item like losing weight in time for your summer holiday. Throughout the site, complex information is presented in manageable chunks, making it very easy to read on screen.

SPECIAL FEATURES

Ask the Expert features Dr Ann Robinson, GP and columnist for The Guardian, children's nurse Hilary Stewart, and smoking cessation specialist Nicola Willis. You can read the daily question as well as answers to previous questions in the archive.

Fitness One of the UK's leading authorities on exercise, Jane Wake, writes for these impressive pages. They include the latest trends in exercise classes, handy workouts for use at home or in a hurry, a fitness test, and general education about exercise. The personal stories of health transformation ('I started to belly dance... and was happy again!') are interesting and inspiring, with links and information provided should you want to take similar action. News includes articles on the latest campaign launches and research findings.

Features are on relatively timeless subjects, such as how a poor diet may affect your health and how to find the right gym for you. They are well done, and are sometimes based on book launches, with an author interview, a review from the site's journalist, an extract, and the opportunity to buy the book at a discount.

Common Conditions is an A-Z of ailments, each posing and answering several questions concisely but thoroughly and providing useful sources of further information.

Natural Health is also known as Think Natural and links you directly to the online vitamin store (see p. 128), which features articles on natural health.

OTHER FEATURES
There are discussion pages, chat rooms, an alphabetical listing of support organisations, and online shopping. Many good links are included within the relevant articles. Other channels in the iCircle network feature other aspects of living such as pregnancy and birth, money, career and relationships – click on Her Money, Ask Anna, Baby World, The Passport (travel) and more.

A relaunch is being planned for this site, but all it really needs is better promotion. It's very well designed, a breeze to use, the information is great and the experts are genuine.

www.handbag.com
Handbag

Overall rating: ★ ★ ★ ★			
Classification:	Ezine	Readability:	★ ★ ★ ★
Updating:	Daily	Content:	★ ★ ★ ★
Navigation:	★ ★ ★ ★	Speed:	★ ★ ★ ★

UK

Handbag is the product of a curious business coupling – the Daily Telegraph and Boots the Chemist – yet this site, which is aimed primarily at women, has emerged with a distinct personality in its own right and is not as fuddy-duddy as its ownership could suggest. From the homepage, select a category from the menu panel at the left, or click on one of the features highlighted in the centre of the page. Once inside each channel, a more specific list of entries will appear in the left-hand menu panel.

SPECIAL FEATURES

Health and Beauty is a comprehensive channel featuring health news, complementary therapies, health issues, healthy eating, patient information, a medical dictionary, and shopping pages. Contributors include Dr Sarah Brewer on complementary medicine, and on conventional treatments, Dr Chris Brown, a GP for 17 years with special interests in womens' health and teenage health education. There is a good Ask the Experts facility plus the Let's Talk message board. Health News addresses the latest research and health product developments, and is lead by Health Scout reporters who point you to further articles on the web and books on related issues. The complementary therapies pages include general articles on treatments like herbalism and aromatherapy, plus news-led pieces on specific products. The self-treatment guide to Bach flower remedies is useful but would be improved by the addition of a facility to search by flower treatment. A click on healthy eating takes you to the food and drink channel – after you've read Roz Denny's advice on counting calories, how to dry-fry and buying olive oil, re-choose the Health and Beauty channel from the pull-down menu if you want to head back there. There is also an extensive online library of patient information leaflets about various conditions. It includes lists of UK self-help groups and simple anatomical diagrams.

Sport and Fitness includes news, features, Ask the Experts, archived articles, and discussion sections, amongst others. Features includes pieces by regular contributor Carolan Brown on exercise and Peter Cohen on slimming, with subjects typically including choice of exercise and high-protein diets. Subjects would benefit by having a more topical slant, with an archive of previous articles. Sports expertise is supplied by Liz Taplin, with Simon Harrison on the specific subject of martial arts. Dr Jeremy Sims is the site authority on mind-body health issues and can be emailed for advice in the Health Chat section, which also features some good archived articles that veer towards beauty and complementary therapy issues.

OTHER FEATURES

A variety of links are included in each channel, and there is also information on careers, education, entertainment, family, fashion, finance, home and garden, motoring, and more.

This handbag may not be jam-packed with celebrities, but the contributors are authoritative and offer much sound advice and information. It's a pleasure to visit.

www.hfonline.co.uk
Health and Fitness Magazine

Overall rating: ★ ★ ★ ★ ★			
Classification:	Magazine	Readability:	★ ★ ★ ★
Updating:	Weekly	Content:	★ ★ ★ ★ ★
Navigation:	★ ★ ★ ★ ★	Speed:	★ ★ ★ ★ ★

UK

Health and Fitness magazine is the UK's leading title for active women and those who would like to be so. Although aimed at general consumers, it is highly respected by professionals in the health and fitness trade because it is not as beauty-oriented as many of its superficial competitors. The site has a fun design with images of girls leaping everywhere, but it can be hard to read the white writing from a pale blue background. The homepage offers several entry points, with menu strips along the top and right-hand side of the screen, and latest features highlighted in the centre. Alternatively, you can search the site by keyword from the box at the top left.

SPECIAL FEATURES

Diary features dance arts, fitness and cooking events around the UK on a weekly basis and provides contact details.

Preview covers the latest book and video releases in the areas of health, exercise, nutrition, self-help, and complementary therapies.

News is updated weekly and features an archive of previous reports.

Forum allows you to post a question or message to other visitors. This section is well-attended and there seems to be a particular enthusiasm for running.

Buyer's Guide offers terrestrial addresses, phone numbers, and email addresses of various businesses around the UK. Whether you need a supplier of exercise gear, Pilates classes, or a health farm, this is the place to come.

Features is a large section with lengthy, in-depth consideration of issues such as vitamin supplementation, why running is the best exercise for cardiovascular health, how to recognise good training shoes, and how to get a gym-style workout at home.

Health Update includes a brief current news story plus a selection of links to sites such as the NHS. Other pages are run along similar lines, including Frontlines, Fitness Matters, Food Matters, and Mind & Body.

Register offers fortnightly emails from personal trainer Jamie Forman as well as the opportunity to win a Reebok exercise cycle.

OTHER FEATURES

Visitor's poll, site search, subscriptions, information about the magazine, and book sales through WH Smith. Links are well chosen and are featured within the pages devoted to each subject area, which is a useful approach.

Fans of the magazine will find little new here other than community interaction, but for those not familiar with the down-to-earth, informative approach of Health and Fitness, this is definitely a site to bookmark. You don't have to be an exercise freak either...in fact, they'll tell you why you shouldn't be.

---

www.phys.com
Phys

Overall rating: ★ ★ ★ ★ ★			
Classification:	Magazine	**Readability:**	★ ★ ★ ★
Updating:	Weekly	**Content:**	★ ★ ★ ★
Navigation:	★ ★ ★	**Speed:**	★ ★ ★ ★

US

A lively site from the US containing content from the Condé Nast range of US women's magazines. Articles come from the superb Women's Sports and Fitness, and also Self, Allure, Glamour, Vogue and Mademoiselle. From the homepage, choose from the menu strip along the top of the screen or click on one of the featured articles or tools on the centre of the screen – it's very busy, with almost too much to choose from.

SPECIAL FEATURES

Fitness includes advice on exercise execution, motivational strategies, several recommended workout programmes, a database of sports and activities, injury database and stretching guide, plus more. The excellent quizzes can help you find the right sport for your personality, assess your metabolism, or analyse the best way to help you stick to an exercise programme.

Nutrition information and advice comes from the experts at prestigious Tufts University, amongst others. This section also includes an encyclopaedic nutrition reference section, dietary self-analysis tools, forums, and features on specific aspects of healthy eating such as vitamin C intake. Eating Right is an excellent archive of articles, such as how to fat-proof your fridge, eat right at each stage of life, increase your soy intake, and avoid the traps of fad diet books. The Nutritional Rx offers dietary advice for different ailments, for example anaemia. Wheel of Portion is an amusing game that helps you understand and calculate appropriate serving sizes for each food group.

Weight Loss brings elements from other parts of the site together in a section devoted to smart eating for size reduction rather than the latest con. It is divided into five main sections helping you to assess yourself, set goals, eat right, get fit, and stay on track – you select the articles you want to view from the pull-down menus for each section. Also here is the Snack Bandit, which explains, through the use of a fruit machine, what you would have to do in order to work off a serving of your favourite treat.

Women's Sports and Fitness magazine covers all the latest thinking in health and fitness research and demonstrates how to apply it to real life. Columnists include Gabrielle Reece, the famed model-cum-beach volleyball star, and US fitness pro Kathy Kaehler.

Self magazine is more glitzy than WS&F. Here you'll find tips from world-famous fitness queen Kathy Smith, plus interactive diet and fitness programs, quizzes, and motivational strategies. The slide shows are an irritating gimmick: they can be speeded up or slowed down, but they are single pictures, not step-by-step instructions for doing exercises.

Experts include the site's own weight-loss coach, nutritionist Terri Browne, plus Molly Fox, an authority on yoga. They each answer several questions a week posted by site visitors, and previous queries are archived.

OTHER FEATURES

News, Breast Health Center, Forums, Horoscopes, Subscriptions.

Phys is an interesting and fun place to visit. Repurposed content can make a dull website when one is familiar with the original publication, but that's not the case here as many of the magazines supplying features are not widely available in the UK.

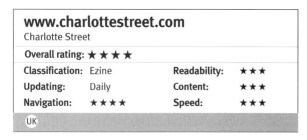

www.charlottestreet.com
Charlotte Street

Overall rating: ★ ★ ★ ★			
Classification:	Ezine	**Readability:**	★ ★ ★
Updating:	Daily	**Content:**	★ ★ ★
Navigation:	★ ★ ★ ★	**Speed:**	★ ★ ★

UK

The tone of Charlotte Street is that of an upmarket tabloid newspaper, and indeed, some of the text comes from Daily Mail writers. The site was heavily advertised when it first launched but was slow to take off as it was more technologically advanced than the computers of the target audience. Viewing the site requires Flash 4. It is not necessary to take out membership, but it's free, and exclusive offers are promised in return, as well as the ability to post questions on the message boards. To enter, click on the yellow and black arrow icon. When the main page appears, choose from the menu panel at the top left of the screen – the subsections of each channel will appear as you move your cursor over them. Alternatively click on one of the features highlighted at the centre of the page. You can directly access the message boards by clicking at the bottom left of the screen

SPECIAL FEATURES

Babies and Family Several health-related issues are covered in this section which is divided into pregnancy and babies, children, and education. Typical subjects are teenage sex, time management for working mothers, whether mobile phones are a particular danger to children, fertility issues, and natural ways to prepare for childbirth.

Look Good Feel Great Although some fashion articles are included here, this channel is predominately about leading a healthier lifestyle. The section features an online nutritionist and covers a fair amount of sport and exercise news, particularly with regard to walking and running events, and women's sports – indeed, it is more about sport than gym-oriented exercise, which makes a refreshing change. Broader health issues covered include HRT, vitamin supplements, and seasonal subjects like hayfever.

Home and Shopping This channel has a food section that often features articles about healthy eating and reports on food trends and research.

Factfiles are included within each channel but can be accessed separately from the menu panel. This section is potentially good but the reference material suffers from oversimplification. You will most likely have heard or read similar health and fitness information before.

OTHER FEATURES

News, weather, horoscopes, work and money, love and marriage, leisure and freetime, feedback. The message boards are well attended and friendly.

Although not as superficial as its launch advertising campaign may have implied, Charlotte Street's editorial coverage is nevertheless a little lightweight compared to its competitors. However, if you prefer healthy living information that is easy to digest and not too worthy, this site is on the right track, and there is a good sense of community in the chat sections.

www.beme.com
BeMe

Overall rating: ★ ★ ★			
Classification:	Magazine	**Readability:**	★ ★
Updating:	Monthly	**Content:**	★ ★ ★
Navigation:	★ ★	**Speed:**	★ ★

UK

The overly funky design of this site belies the fact that much of its content seems to be derived from relatively mainstream magazines such as Woman, Woman's Weekly, Woman's Realm, and Essentials. The site has undergone a massive redesign since its launch, but it is still has some way to go to be truly effective. From the slow-to-load homepage, click on the picture of Björk, also known as Section Three or Home Life. Once in that channel, a menu panel on the left offers a selection of rather precious headings including Nurture (children, not plants), Grow (plants, not children), Love, and so on.

SPECIAL FEATURES

Thrive is the main health section of the site and features articles from the website's correspondents as well as stories from IPC magazines. Dieting, alternative therapies, vitamins and supplements are typical subjects, and the quality of the writing and advice given varies greatly.

Eat (in) contains more reused material from the magazines, and although it doesn't have a particular health focus, you may find articles describing the many varieties of salad leaves now available in stores or new chicken recipes to try.

Shop is a series of links to companies such as Think Natural and Nutravida (see pp. 128 and 120). There is a food shopping section here, too.

Advice and Info 'This incredibly valuable resource area is living proof of our commitment to making your life as easy as possible'. Perhaps a little overstated? Choose Health and Medical from the pull-down menu here and you can browse an A-Z of common ailments with advice on recognising symptoms and what to do when ill.

OTHER FEATURES

Other channels include News, Consumer Affairs (this is good and put together by someone with a wicked sense of humour), Culture and Trends, Entertainment, and a facility to personalise the site to reflect your own interests. The chat sections of each channel are named after the rooms of a house such as kitchen in the consumer section and bedroom in Home Life.

The design smothers what is at times good content, and it's unclear for whom this site is intended – trendoids who might appreciate the stylised elements aren't going to thrill to editorial gleaned from Woman's Realm.

www.channelhealth.net
Channel Health

Overall rating: ★ ★ ★		
Classification: Ezine	**Readability:**	★ ★ ★ ★
Updating: Monthly	**Content:**	★ ★ ★
Navigation: ★ ★ ★	**Speed:**	★ ★ ★

UK

At first Channel Health looks too stylised for its own good, a swirl of funky but obscure symbols appears and moving your cursor over them to reveal the pictures clarifies little. But then you see that the menu panel down the left-hand side of the screen features Hazel Courteney, one of Britain's top writers on alternative health strategies, which must mean it's worth further investigation, at least once. Other experts are Doctor Robert Lefever, a specialist in addictive behaviour, and Eddie and Debbie Shapiro, specialists in relaxation.

In every channel we reviewed the lead story was about the availability of Channel Health on television and how you could become a subscriber to Sky Digital (it's so easy!). When we clicked on 'Talk to Hazel', expecting the opportunity to pose a question, we were told about a premium-rate phone line on which we could hear Hazel talk about her near-death experience for 50p per minute. Very off-putting.

SPECIAL FEATURES

His Her lives to 'support and celebrate the sensual, life-giving, charming, erotic and gorgeous person you are'. It's a disparate blend of general short features, women and men only sections, plus sex, pregnancy and diet. The tone is middle-market tabloid, with stories prompted by recent book releases. It looks as though there must be loads of content but in fact many of the articles in this channel are also to be found elsewhere on the site.

Grey Matters has a logo seemingly inspired by the Two Fat Ladies – a couple raring to go on a motorcycle. The Pillow Talk section turned out to be advice on sleeping, but there were articles elsewhere about sex for retired people. The Diet Advice section was on eating a raw food diet.

THC is 'teen health club', supposedly, and included an article entitled 'Sex – Making the First Move', which had also been published in the His Her adult section, where the reader was transported when clicking on the feature. Here too was an article discussing the pros and cons of marijuana and one on why dance music makes you horny. One presumes this channel is intended for people around or over the age of consent, young adults maybe, not 'teens' as in 'thirteen'.

Tots 2 Teens is about parenting.

Pleasure Principle combines pop psychology and relationships counselling with eating, feng shui beauty and

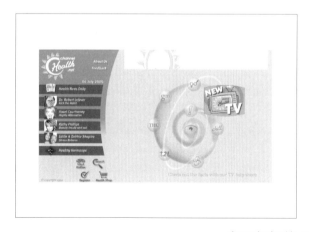

tips on addictive behaviour. A somewhat arbitrary combination.

Chill Out includes getaway ideas, stress-busting music, dream analysis, gentle exercise. Not bad.

Fix It is the medically-oriented channel but includes space clearing and pet health.

OTHER FEATURES

Health news, healthy horoscope, shopping, separate channels for each expert

Overly commercial, pretentiously designed and at times ill-judged in its editorial content, Channel Health does have a few good features in its archive, but other sites have the edge as information resources.

OTHER SITES OF INTEREST

Shape Magazine
www.shapemag.com
Shape is one of the world's best lifestyle magazines for active women and is licensed to publishers in several countries around the world. This site is the home of the mother of all Shapes, the American edition, headed by the guru-esque editorial director Barbara S Harris (the thinking-woman's fitness leader, if ever there was one) and world-renowned weight lifting megastar Joe Weider, who is the publisher. The site features extracts from the current US edition – always authoritative, thought-provoking, and at the leading edge of fitness and healthy lifestyle theories. Some original site content would be nice though....

Thrive Online
www.thriveonline.com
An ezine extolling the virtues of a healthy lifestyle, Thrive Online is one of the better known American sites and covers all key areas including nutrition and medical health issues. Perhaps its key attribute, however, is Karen Voight, an American fitness superstar who has achieved worldwide recognition through being just so damn good. Here is the place to come when you want to read her advice on common problems or begin a Voight workout plan. For the complete novice, there is an excellent structured walking programme.

iVillage
www.ivillage.com
Our general impression of this site, having subscribed to its newsletters for some time, is that it's very much like a magazine for young women. There is a large dieting section, which is always ready to consider the latest trend on the health book market, and plenty of celebrity-oriented features.

Food Fitness
www.foodfitness.org.uk
This site is aimed at people who have never given much thought to what a healthy lifestyle might involve or require. It's attractively designed and well-written, using the example of two 'typical' families – one unhealthy group that sits or lies in front of the TV as often as possible eating takeaways, and one with an achieveably active lifestyle. The point is to show you how to become more like the latter and there are some good tips here for increasing your basic level of everyday activity, which plays a key role in your overall level of fitness.

Chapter 4

special diets

Never has Western culture been more aware of what it eats. Our daily food choices combine to have a major impact on our health; they affect our size and shape, certainly, but they can also increase the risk of developing fatal conditions like cancer and heart disease. Obesity, for example, is a contributing factor in many illnesses, from comparatively minor ailments such as joint pain and feet trouble to high-profile killer diseases.

It pays to achieve and maintain a healthy weight, but you don't have to pay through the nose to do it. There are many excellent free services on the internet to help you eat well and choose food appropriately, whether you are overweight, underweight, diabetic, vegetarian, allergic to wheat, or simply looking for a few healthy recipes.

Scaremongers like to pedal the notion that there are thousands of dodgy companies on the internet promising the impossible and charging the incredible. Such stories make good copy for newspapers. The truth is, however, that if you want reliable advice on weight management, healthy eating, or special diets, there is absolutely no reason for you to go anywhere near those unreputable sites.

When visiting the sites recommended here, be sure to distinguish between the information presented by the professionals and the opinions of the general public posted on message boards. Although message boards can be a good way of making friends and giving and receiving support in your healthy eating endeavours, they are not reputable sources of information, even when well moderated by a responsible company.

www.cyberdiet.com
Cyberdiet

Overall rating: ★ ★ ★ ★ ★

Classification:	Information	**Readability:**	★ ★ ★
Updating:	Daily	**Content:**	★ ★ ★ ★ ★
Navigation:	★ ★ ★ ★	**Speed:**	★ ★ ★ ★

US

Part of the Mediconsult health network, this is one of the internet's most respected health sites and is full of sound advice on achieving and maintaining a healthy weight. It is as relevant to underweight as overweight people. The jam-packed homepage features seasonal and community features at the centre of the page, with tools and main channels listed down the side in coloured panels.

SPECIAL FEATURES

Self Assessment offers several tools to help analyse and monitor your health. It covers nutrition profiles as well as body mass index, waist-to-hip ratio and risk assessment.

Diet & Nutrition covers various aspects of eating, such as recipe makeovers or how to dine out without too much damage to your waistline. It also assesses which diet books have sound theories and which are the cons. The recipes have a strong American bias, although British visitors can still gain a lot from visiting. The easy-to-use daily food planner allows you to choose recipes and dishes to fit in with your calorie requirements (which you would have analysed in the self-assessment section).

Exercise & Fitness offers motivational tips, advice on choosing the right exercise for you, and a tool for assessing how much activity you are doing.

Support & Motivation is based very much on contributions from other site visitors. In many respects this section works well – success stories are always a popular feature in magazines and newspapers and this is true on the web too. However it's not all jolly: indeed, it can be quite heart-breaking to read about the terrible extremes some visitors have felt driven to. Impressively, many of the support facilities are broken down into categories such as discussion groups for teenagers, people with more than 100lb to lose, or people who are trying to give up smoking without putting weight on. Also here is a fun Meditation Room that allows you to download relaxation exercises – after all, stress is a common cause of over eating.

Resource Centre branches out from food and exercise to cover other health issues such as depression and diet, treating diabetes, pregnancy, HIV, cancer and digestive disorders.

Newsletter gives regular updates of additions to the site, plus notification of live chats from the Cyberdiet hosts. Links are provided to articles which cover a broad remit: typical features might include a cheery piece on seasonal produce, news analysis of the latest dietary recommendations, advice on seeking psychiatric help for children, and the pros and cons of particular dieting products.

OTHER FEATURES
Ask the Experts, Polls.

A very well-conceived site with much input from the site hosts and visitors. People who are extremely overweight or very isolated will find a degree of positive support and community not generally available elsewhere.

www.mynutrition.co.uk
My Nutrition

Overall rating: ★ ★ ★ ★ ★			
Classification:	Information	Readability:	★ ★ ★ ★ ★
Updating:	Monthly	Content:	★ ★ ★ ★
Navigation:	★ ★ ★ ★	Speed:	★ ★ ★ ★

UK

Set up in 1998 by Health Co Ltd, My Nutrition aims to help individuals make adjustments to their diet and assess which vitamins or minerals are needed. You'll have to wait while the site does its fancy flashing words bit at the beginning, but eventually this stops and a flower shape is revealed with each petal being a subject channel. You simply click on the one you want, and as you move the cursor over each petal, an explanatory paragraph pops up explaining what you'll find within.

SPECIAL FEATURES

My Consultation is a free service, and so it should be because it's not anything new, just repurposed content from Patrick Holford's Optimum Nutrition books. If you have not encountered these before, you may find this section useful; however, health enthusiasts will find little here that they have not read before. A very general list of recommended vitamins and supplements is given at the end of the interactive quiz along with basic dietary guidelines (the ones they reckon are particular to you are highlighted in bold). Their speedy response to subsequent questions regarding why some supplements were recommended and not others was impressive, and it was explained that recommendations were made on the assumption that dietary recommendations will be followed to the letter. This section should be improved by forthcoming changes.

My Library is better than the name suggests, and is the basic background articles you need to understand good nutrition. Covered here are the basic principles of healthy eating, taking supplements, and health at various stages of life. The Good Food section within Eating Well features reasons to buy organic food, superfoods for the 21st century, and a sample week's menu. Foods that we've forgotten is a silly name for what is quite an informative piece (but again, repurposed content). Cooking methods discusses the pros and cons of deep-frying, stir-frying, microwaving, and so on.

My News features short monthly articles from Patrick Holford on timely issues. On a recent visit, tips were included on how to boost immunity and kill colds, along with a piece on the dropping sperm count of the British male, and advice from Ian Marber, author of a book called The Food Doctor.

My Conditions is an A–Z of ailments with natural remedies such as herbal ointments, aromatherapy oils, and diet and supplement advice. We liked this, although it is a simple reference section – it contained many good ideas not found on other sites.

My Stuff allows you to record purchases and results of your 'consultation quiz' in a private area accessible by password. The company has plans to expand this facility.

OTHER FEATURES

Shopping.

Although initially put off by the site's enthusiasm for prescribing and selling vitamin supplements, on subsequent visits we grew to like My Nutrition. Hiding behind the glossy façade is some good information and useful articles. What would really improve this site, however, is more original content from a wider variety of nutrition practitioners.

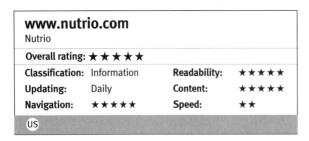

www.nutrio.com
Nutrio

Overall rating: ★ ★ ★ ★ ★		
Classification: Information	**Readability:**	★ ★ ★ ★ ★
Updating: Daily	**Content:**	★ ★ ★ ★ ★
Navigation: ★ ★ ★ ★ ★	**Speed:**	★ ★

US

There's an impressive team of experts behind this weight loss community site including several senior dietitians, doctors and sports specialists. The site is scattered with brief but enthusiastic testimonials from visitors. The main channels are listed down the left-hand side of the screen with another menu strip at the top of the page. Several features are highlighted on the homepage, which requires a lot of scrolling to take in all the information. The keyword search facility is on the lower left.

SPECIAL FEATURES

Weight Loss Program This is also known as MyNutrio and Weight Loss Wizard and is free. You answer a series of 19 questions so that your personalised program may be calculated, and you are then given some feedback on your answers. This is one of the best versions of this type of thing we have found on the web – it really was personalised to our answers and our only criticism, apart from the general low speed of the site, was that the calorie amounts recommended for weight loss were a little too strict – you may want to add a couple of hundred calories if you have a lot of weight to lose or are active. Your eating plan then appears on the homepage of the site on a daily basis once you've logged in, and you can click on the links beneath it to check out the weekly menu plan, exercise plan, record your progress, and so on. Be

aware, too, that some ingredient substitutions for things like non-fat cream cheese may need to be made in the recipes.

Features are highlighted at the centre of the page and typical content includes 'what we mean by healthy shopping', 'life as fitness', 'controlling cravings with exercise' and anger management techniques. Click on the More link to be presented with more options. Beginners will find this section particularly useful. The articles are informative but not too long, and there are some great ideas for healthy living such as 'cross training is as easy as choosing a new activity', 'correct posture can make you look about 10–15 pounds lighter instantly' and advice on how to fit regular exercise into a busy schedule. There are links to other relevant articles at the base of each one, and every time you click on a new subject a new window opens, which you will either find useful or it will drive you mad, depending on the size of your screen.

Daily News is the place for topical stories and response to new research findings. 'A Woman's Workout is Work' has boffins telling us nothing we didn't know already, girls: they found that 95 per cent of women over 40 get their exercise from doing household chores. Some content comes from news agencies such as HealthSCOUT. Click through to the archive for a list of other newsy articles – there's plenty of interest here, including broader health issues such as the dangers of trampolining for children and how sugar placebos are actually reasonable cures for serious problems.

Nutrition 'Are you fat phobic?' they ask here, with the aim to make visitors realise that while the fat content of foods is important when dieting, calories are important too, and cutting down fat too much can cause bingeing. A memorable statistic was that one teaspoon of oil contains 45 calories but so does one cup of raw salad vegetables. Also here are steps to a skinnier, healthier kitchen, tips for eating healthily on the go when you're vegetarian, and ways to give your children a nutritious start in life. There are plenty of archived articles, so you will have plenty of reason to keep coming back here.

Fitness Keeping fit when travelling, advice for running your first 10K race, the key to exercising regularly, why you should never skip your warm-up and 'The Executive's Guide to Deskercise' are typical subjects in this article-led channel.

Mind/Body Discover here how to stay positive and focused while dieting, how to say 'no' to being too thin, why weighing yourself more than once a week could sabotage your efforts, how to cope with comments that you would be pretty if only you lost weight, plus other interesting health issues such as how to improve your sleep and keep your brain functioning at optimal levels.

Tools All the usual suspects are here – a healthy weight to height chart, how to calculate your body mass index and target heart rate, a calorie burn guide explaining how much energy various sports and activities use up, a food analyser with the nutritional content of individual foods and drinks. The Fast Food Facts section is dominated by American takeaway chains, but some of the information is relevant to UK visitors – such as full nutritional breakdowns for McDonalds, Pizza Hut and KFC products, so if you fell off the wagon you know how much it hurt.

References includes the USDA's healthy eating pyramids, details of how to understand America's nutrition labels and other wording on packaging, plus comprehensive sections explaining all you need to know about vitamins and minerals.

Community There are separate message boards for nutrition, fitness and mind/body, with a choice of subjects in each and all are very well attended. The Starting Place for new participants in the nutrition section is obviously popular, but there's also a recipe exchange, a board called

Moving on Up for students and young professionals, plus the Dr's Orders board focusing on the progress of one particular member. Motivation is the key subject in the exercise message boards while the mind/body boards cover emotional eating, a section for those with more than 100 pounds to lose, one for those over forty and an 'I did it!' board for taking a bow.

OTHER FEATURES

Poll, nutrition quiz, newsletter, send to a friend.

Apart from working a teensy bit slowly, and their ruthless calorie restriction, this is a very fine site indeed, and one you will be keen to come back to for support and information in any weight-loss efforts.

www.nutritiouslygourmet.com
Nutritiously Gourmet

Overall rating: ★ ★ ★ ★ ★			
Classification: Information		**Readability:**	★ ★ ★ ★
Updating: Weekly		**Content:**	★ ★ ★ ★ ★
Navigation: ★ ★ ★ ★		**Speed:**	★ ★ ★

US

This charming, but unfortunately slow-to-load site offers a monthly menu with well-written recipes, photos, and nutritional analyses. Host Jane A Rubey holds a Master's degree in public health (nutrition) and is a registered dietitian in the US. She also taught nutrition and food science courses at the California Culinary Academy in San Francisco. 'One might think I'm trying to take the fun out of eating,' she says. 'Quite the contrary. I am trying to take advantage of the information we have which allows us to build our health so that we can truly have fun, not just while eating, but in the whole of life. And working to rebuild the environment and ensure a sustainable future seems to be an important part of that larger picture.' The site is very easy to navigate and read; however, the pages are way too long, and a lot of scrolling is required.

SPECIAL FEATURES

Menus/Recipes   Jane aims to combine the latest in nutritional knowledge with delicious recipes using seasonal produce. The basic premise is that each menu should be creative but nutritionally balanced to contain 20 per cent fat, 10 per cent protein and 70 per cent carbs, primarily starches. Recent visits have seen Jane taking a Mexican theme, with fish tostadas, yogurt cheese, guacamole, and salsa verde. Another typical menu would be lentil burger with trimmings and strawberry mousse cake with strawberry sauce. Notes on the menus discuss issues such as the provenance of

ingredients, and alternatives to those suggested. Within this section there is a glossary of menu terms and ingredients to refer to. Scroll down underneath the menus to read the recipes.

Nutrition Basics   Much of Nutritiously Gourmet's work is based on The China Study, an ongoing nutrition research project that has highlighted the relationship between disease and poor Western eating habits. Extensive information is provided here, addressing the components of foods as well as specific diseases. Jane A Rubey brings in other research, recommendations from the USDA, and a variety of dietary pyramids for different cultures, including one for vegetarians. This is comprehensive, informative, and excellent – apart from all that damn scrolling!

Seasonal Produce   Information on organic foods and sustainable agriculture is found here. There is a calendar with a key denoting whether produce is new season, at peak or winding down. Obviously it's American, but Brits may find some stuff here of interest since we're all in the northern hemisphere.

Nutrition News   Timely facts and summaries of the latest research (with references provided) are featured here. Interesting items on a recent visit included a list of 12 healthy eating do's and don'ts, including suggestions to eat plant-only dinners at least three times a week, news that meat intake has been linked to increased risk of particular cancers, and news that eggs are okay for most people (as is coffee – hurrah!).

'Cooking with Nutritiously Gourmet beats eating an apple a day!' they claim, and we have to agree. What a shame that we are limited to just one menu each month from this brilliant dietitian-cook.

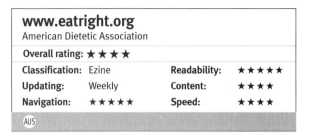

www.eatright.org
American Dietetic Association

Overall rating: ★ ★ ★ ★			
Classification:	Ezine	Readability:	★ ★ ★ ★ ★
Updating:	Weekly	Content:	★ ★ ★ ★
Navigation:	★ ★ ★ ★ ★	Speed:	★ ★ ★ ★

AUS

The American Dietetic Association's site is designed for health professionals and consumers. It's colourful and easy to navigate as well as authoritative and simple to understand. On the homepage, click on one of the cartoon icons to choose your department.

SPECIAL FEATURES

Nutrition Resources is divided into two lists, one for consumers and one for professionals. Scroll down to the section you want and click on the highlighted features. New additions to this section are marked with a red logo. The section includes excerpts from ADA-recommended books such as Dieting for Dummies, plus advice on implementing the dietary guidelines illustrated by the food dietary pyramid. There are daily nutrition and healthy lifestyle tips. Advice from the ADA is not as geared towards counting calories and fat-grams as most other sites. Although weight loss and maintenance is a concern, this is more about healthy eating and living in general, about getting the balance of foods right in your diet.

In the News aims to reveal 'the science behind the sound bites' and to explain clearly the truth about headlines and health scares reported in the media by pointing readers to ADA resources. Typical coverage could be trans-fatty acids, food safety and hygiene, diet drugs, and low-carb, high-protein diets. A key component of this section is Ten Red

Flags of Junk Science, found on the right of the screen. It's an excellent, highly sensible tool to help you recognise false claims and cons yourself.

Government Affairs is accessed by clicking on the drawing of the White House. It is a useful section for those with a broader professional or deep amateur interest in health issues. Here the ADA talks about its latest liaisons with the US Government and its various departments, providing some insight into the regulations or recommendations that may soon be affecting us.

OTHER FEATURES

Member services, Press Room for journalists, Marketplace, and more.

Look here if you are interested in healthy eating or weight management but would like to try a non-dieting approach.

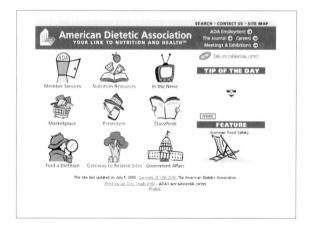

www.caloriecontrol.org
Calorie Control Council

Overall rating: ★ ★ ★ ★			
Classification: Information		**Readability:**	★ ★ ★ ★
Updating: Weekly		**Content:**	★ ★ ★
Navigation: ★ ★ ★ ★		**Speed:**	★ ★ ★ ★

US

Although designed to look like a ten-year-old low-cal ready-meal box, this site nevertheless has several useful tools and is jam-packed with common sense. The Calorie Control Council seems to be an alliance of companies with particular interest in producing low-calorie as well as low-fat foods, and promoting their inclusion in daily diets. If your screen is small, you will need to scroll down past the headline and pictures of cream cakes to find the entry points to the site. There is a keyword search facility at the bottom of the page.

SPECIAL FEATURES

News Net highlights the week's top news stories regarding health and weight control.

Let's Get Physical demonstrates the need to be active when it comes to weight control and maintenance. As they say, 'It's bad enough that more Americans than ever are overweight. Is the problem being compounded by an over-emphasis on only one method of fixing it?' That method is, of course, dieting and the answer is yes. There are tips here for setting fitness goals, and the US Surgeon General's Report on why a sedentary lifestyle is hazardous to health.

How to Win by Losing is a brief guide to weight control. This section is broken down into short pieces that address more than calorie intake; also included are ten tips to help you reshape behaviour, motivational tips, and advice on

maintenance. This section emphasises the importance of physical activity in achieving a healthy weight too.

Calories Still Count sounds almost like a plea! This section argues the need to control calorie intake despite the focus over the last decade or so on the importance of limiting fat in the diet. As the article points out, it doesn't matter if a product is labelled low-calorie, low-fat and low-sugar, you can't eat ten packs of it without suffering consequences.

Light Living takes an in-depth look at artificial sweeteners and fat replacers, and aims to address arguments for and against them. The section takes each major brand in turn and reports on research results. Although it aims to be balanced, there does seem to be a conflict of interest. This section may set your mind at rest if you are worried about, for example, eating aspartame-flavoured diet products.

Calculators The enhanced calorie calculator allows you to keep a list of what you have eaten during the day, with nutrition information analysed, as opposed to the regular calorie calculator which simply provides the nutritional breakdown of various foods. Also here is an exercise calculator to help you analyse how many calories you expend performing various activities. The body mass index calculator helps establish how over- or underweight you are and whether or not you are consequently at risk of developing health problems.

Recipes includes meal plans created by dietitians who won the Calorie Control Council's healthy menu contest. Dishes include chocolate custard, raspberry-swirl peach soup, orange spice coffee cake, loin of pork with tart cherry sauce, and more.

OTHER FEATURES

Newsletter, monthly feature, What the Labels Mean, FAQs, What's New, Trends and Statistics, The Press Room, Fat

Replacers, Companies and Products, and a section for health professionals and educators.

The stance is generally pro-artificial sweeteners and fat replacers, so enthusiastic consumers of natural foods and organics won't be happy here, but if the invention of low-fat, low-cal diet chocolate mousses has made all the difference to your weight loss efforts, this is a good site for you.

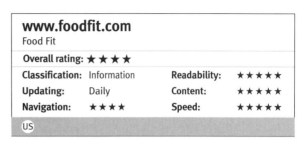

www.foodfit.com
Food Fit

Overall rating: ★ ★ ★ ★			
Classification:	Information	**Readability:**	★ ★ ★ ★ ★
Updating:	Daily	**Content:**	★ ★ ★ ★ ★
Navigation:	★ ★ ★ ★	**Speed:**	★ ★ ★ ★ ★

US

Ellen Haas, the founder of this site, has impressive credentials as a public health advocate; she has spent more than 20 years running government nutrition programmes in the US, overseen a revision of the school lunch programme, and been elected five times as president of the Consumer Federation of America. The aim of the site is to help the public lead a healthier life through good food and active living. The lively and highly illustrated homepage can give the impression that there is little here of benefit to British visitors, packed as it is with American products and stories. However, it is worth persevering. To move to the useful information, click on the channels listed along the base of the banner at the top of the screen.

SPECIAL FEATURES

Healthy Eating is a huge topic and subsequently this channel is divided into several smaller sections, including Season's Pick, Foods in the News, guides to rice and beans, and more. Our last visit saw an article on summer squashes, their nutritional benefits, the varieties available and recipes. You could learn more about the cancer-fighting properties of tea, tomatoes, and garlic, refer to the seasonal fruit and vegetable chart, and find out what the site's experts have to say about biotech foods. There is a link here to Food Fit's 'seven step plan for healthy living', plus an archive of previously published material.

Healthy Cooking Food Fit has the support of a large network of American chefs including some of the top names in the business, several of whom have contributed recipes to the site in sections such as Chefs@Home. It's not about fancy cooking however; you will find plenty of quick and easy recipes here, plus useful tips to add a twist to your regular meals. The Recipe Revue features makeovers of down-home dishes such as frankfurters and beans. There are Menus for the Week from Chef Bonnie who provides useful advance preparation instructions to make everything run as smoothly as possible.

Tools There are several offered. First take your Food Fit profile, which requires site registration, and is a series of questions to determine your nutritional strengths and weaknesses – recipes are then offered that fit your needs. Also here are a healthy weight calculator, a calorie burner calculator, a menu planner, a pantry stocker and a tool to help you establish how low you need to cook foods for safety.

Fitness is a great section acknowledging that food and fitness go hand in hand. It covers cardiovascular, resistance and flexibility exercises, plus fitness trends such as meditation. There is plenty here for those new to exercise, and thought-provoking articles for those already interested in fitness, such as a look at why swimmers may sometimes need to eat differently from runners.

Links to food and nutrition sites, chefs and restaurants, plus exercise sources.

OTHER FEATURES

Marketplace for product sales.

This is definitely one to bookmark for a tasty spin on dieting and healthy living information.

www.living-foods.com
Living and Raw Foods

Overall rating: ★ ★ ★			
Classification:	Homepage	**Readability:**	★ ★ ★ ★
Updating:	Varies	**Content:**	★ ★ ★ ★
Navigation:	★ ★ ★ ★	**Speed:**	★ ★ ★ ★

US

The aim of this community-style site about eating raw foods is to 're-educate the world about how simple health can be'. They aim to do so by providing information and support rather than working to convince people of anything. The site is very easy to navigate: the menu strip on the left is for frequent users with features highlighted on the grid at the centre of the page. First-time visitors are shown what it's all about immediately – just click on the link at the top of the grid.

SPECIAL FEATURES

FAQ explains what is meant by the terms 'living and raw foods'. The key is the presence of enzymes which are destroyed by heating food. The proponents of this diet believe that these are the life force or energy of food and help the digestion. Living foods differ a little from raw in the way that a beansprout differs from a bean. Eating organically is also an important aspect of this method of eating.

Articles includes information sheets on subjects such as 'Ten advantages of eating raw', 'Is cooked food good for us?', 'Enzymes and longevity', and 'Natural hygiene – what it is and where it came from'. More practical for first-time visitors is the piece advising how to make the transition from a cooked diet to a raw one. The feature on overcoming problems in raw and living foods diets is labelled a must read: 'The reality of raw diets,' says the author Thomas E Bilings, who has been living this way since the 1970s, 'is that many try such diets but very few succeed on them.' Also here are book reviews and articles explaining the differences between the various sub-types of raw food diets, such as liquidarian, fruitarian, sproutarian. 'The Ins and Outs of Nut Processing' explains why some may not be as raw as you think.

Recipes claims to be the largest online collection of living and raw food recipes. It is divided into types of dishes such as drinks, entrées and side dishes, appetizers, cookies and treats, and so on. Visitors are invited to submit. The quick and easy apple pie is made with a crust of ground sunflower seeds, carob, and raisins, plus a filling of pulverised apples, lemon juice, honey and spices, then left to set in the fridge.

In the News is organised by title of original publication rather than date, so the more recent features require scrolling down the page. Here (unusually for an American site), they feature many articles on raw food lifestyle from the British media including Health and Fitness magazine (see p. 70), the Daily Telegraph and Sunday Times.

City Guides aims to make it easy for people to stay raw wherever they are and includes shops, markets, support groups, and so on. Unfortunately, it is difficult to search.

OTHER FEATURES

Community, bookstore, marketplace, chat, personals and much more.

It's clearly a lifestyle as well as a diet, and not something to be taken lightly. But these people are experts in the subject and the site is a good source of reference and support should you be contemplating this way of living.

www.veganchef.com
The Vegan Chef

Overall rating: ★ ★ ★ ★			
Classification:	Enthusiasts	**Readability:**	★ ★ ★ ★
Updating:	Fortnightly	**Content:**	★ ★ ★ ★ ★
Navigation:	★ ★ ★ ★	**Speed:**	★ ★ ★ ★

US

This is a lively and well-designed recipe site from young chef Beverly Lynn Bennett who is committed to developing exciting and original low-fat, vegan menus. The homepage takes a while to come up, but once inside, the stylish graphics are no problem. Click on one of the apples at the left of the page to reach the main sections, or scroll down to read Bev's welcome, her definition of the word vegan, or sign the guestbook. The featured recipes are all on one page, which requires a lot of scrolling.

SPECIAL FEATURES

Recipes On a recent visit we saw Beverly highlighting Mediterranean dishes such as tzatziki made from soy products, wholewheat pittas with sesame seeds, dolmas, tofu feta-style cheese made with miso and other flavourings, plus a baklava. She's certainly inventive and inspirational. Occasionally the recipes need items such as soy soured cream which are not yet available in the UK, but these small problems are the kind of thing most vegans are used to coping with and let's face it, what's the difference between tofu yogurt and tofu soured cream? Beverly publishes around 12 recipes per month, offering a mix of both easy and more involved dishes. The recipe archive is usefully organised by type of dish and they all sound mouth watering: Florentine fennel salad, broccoli allíaglio, tomato and spinach melt sandwich, garbanzo bean and eggplant ragu, sun-dried tomato olive bread, baked tofu masala, and almond cake.

OTHER FEATURES

A biography, and lots of links to other related vegan and vegetarian sites, and health pages such as Ask Dr Weil.

We're sure most people would be happy to eat vegan with Beverly as their personal chef. She uses a great variety of ingredients in fun dishes, many of which make good fare for parties or special dinners, but you will also find simple, stylish soups, salads and dips for everyday eating, and thankfully no preaching. Someone should get this girl a book deal!

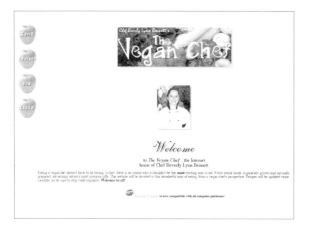

www.vegsoc.org
The Vegetarian Society

Overall rating: ★ ★ ★ ★			
Classification:	Society	Readability:	★ ★ ★ ★
Updating:	Monthly	Content:	★ ★ ★ ★
Navigation:	★ ★ ★ ★	Speed:	★ ★ ★ ★

UK

An ear of corn down the left-hand side of the screen is a fine design choice for this informative site from the UK Vegetarian Society – the world's first and still perhaps the best. As the site demonstrates, the organisation is working towards 'a future where the vegetarian diet is acknowledged as the norm', and to this end talks about much more than what we put in our mouths. The design has improved in recent months: it's now much clearer to read and easier to use, yet remains lively and colourful. Scroll down until beneath the logo if necessary, then click on the icon for each subject heading or use the keyword search facility.

SPECIAL FEATURES

What's New highlights latest additions to the site, plus the Vegetarian Society's current press releases. These may be items promoting vegetarianism generally (such as the annual National Vegetarian Week), a timely recipe suggestion, or the society's latest cookbook. The Local Event section helps you keep up to date and get involved with other enthusiastic vegetarians in your area.

Cordon Vert is a jewel in the Vegetarian Society's crown – the cookery school that offers an impressively diverse range of courses for amateur and professional cooks. Here is class information, plus a large collection of recipes (mainly reproduced from The Vegetarian magazine), many of which are illustrated.

Health and Nutrition includes useful and concise information sheets on a wide variety of subjects. These include individual foods (grains, cheese, nuts and seeds, pulses, and soya), fats and cholesterol, iron, protein, vegan nutrition, vitamin B12, zinc, plus short takes on individual conditions, such as cancers, food poisoning and pesticide residues, heart disease, kidney stones, osteoporosis, and more. Other sections have advice on pregnancy, infants and children, sports and physical activity, and research. Also included here is basic nutrition information from 21st Century Vegetarian, an online version of a small book with an introduction by Sir Paul McCartney, available to buy from the Society. It highlights that although vegetarians can stuff themselves with chocolate and chips, they will not necessarily be doing themselves any good.

New Veggies is a useful starting point for anyone contemplating the change to a vegetarian lifestyle.

OTHER FEATURES

Online store with a fun gift catalogue, book sales, information about animals and the environment, local vegetarian networks, latest press releases from the Society, youth pages, membership information, and links to other vegetarian organisations.

An admirable site that brings together the Vegetarian Society's broad interests very well indeed. It is an excellent source of support and information for lone vegetarians, but may equally cause you to contemplate how many people are today claiming to be vegetarian but not taking it seriously or committing fully. The information and recipes here are useful for such part-timers, but the Society does generally appeal more to those who may be vegetarian for philosophical rather than dietary reasons.

www.vegsource.com
VegSource

Overall rating: ★ ★ ★			
Classification:	Ezine	Readability:	★ ★ ★
Updating:	Daily	Content:	★ ★ ★
Navigation:	★ ★ ★ ★	Speed:	★ ★ ★ ★ ★

US

'Saving the Earth one byte at a time' is the motto of this campaigning online magazine for committed vegetarians. It is particularly good for nutritional information and research on the relationship between meat intake and disease. The homepage is a little confusing because there is so much to see – to view the articles, read the list of subjects from the column at the far right of the screen.

SPECIAL FEATURES

Magazine VegSource's articles do not hesitate to be controversial or a little 'out there'. Rather than settle for features along the lines of 'eat organic, it's good', on a recent visit we found a campaign to maintain high organic standards by exposing weaknesses in the accreditation system. Several of the featured articles reach not only into broader health issues, but ones of philosophy, and many of the authors have PhDs. VegSource does not hesitate to tackle popular subject areas opposing their own beliefs. We found an interesting essay on the current buzz for high protein diets and information on turning vegetarian as a means of beating cancer or heart disease. Several of the contributors are doctors and the past columns are archived in a link at the bottom of the page.

Organic Gardening is a recent addition to the site and includes various tips on dealing with bugs, plant diseases, and composting.

Discussion Boards These are extraordinarily diverse, the key being that rather than discussing vegetarianism, these are for vegetarians discussing subjects of interest to them. Other issues covered home schooling, smoking, parenting, and Star Trek! There is a clubby but educated atmosphere, and several boards are hosted by well-known US experts, such as the highly esteemed Dr Joyce Verdal on keeping fit. FAQ includes queries about cancer, what every vegetarian needs to know, and info about Veg Source.

Recipes The site has its own expert, Chef Deb, to devise menus and dishes for them, and these are highlighted in the semi-regular newsletters. There are several themed options (Veg Starter Kit, Four Food Groups, Healthy Effective Weight Loss) plus a directory of 10,000 recipes on the site – this has doubled in the last six months and will undoubtedly continue to grow.

OTHER FEATURES

Book reviews, live chat, nutritional information, advice for new vegetarians, and much more. There are many links throughout the site – indeed, many of the articles featured are in fact linked.

Well worth visiting for committed vegetarians, plus those who take an interest in serious nutritional information, such as the latest thinking on faddy diets. Even the discussion boards are better and more serious than most. However, while VegSource aims to be open and balanced, the site does seem to suffer from the politicking and backbiting that is sadly all too common amongst those with a professional interest in vegetarianism. The sections where this is the case are invariably highlighted and you can follow the to and fro of the arguing yourself.

www.inside-story.com
The Inside Story

Overall rating: ★ ★ ★			
Classification:	Ezine	Readability:	★ ★ ★ ★
Updating:	Varies	Content:	★ ★ ★ ★ ★
Navigation:	★ ★ ★	Speed:	★ ★ ★

UK

Describing itself as 'the complete resource site for those on special diets or with food allergies and sensitivities', this site includes extracts from the Inside Story magazine founded by Michelle Berriedale-Johnson. The mother of a child with severe food allergies, Michelle has become one of the UK's leading authorities on special dietary needs and food allergies. The categorisation of information can be a little confusing, and it's very slow given the lack of images. You can work from the menu strip at the left side of the screen or the text links in the centre of the homepage. The long text pages need a lot of scrolling and should really be broken down into smaller files.

SPECIAL FEATURES

What are Food Allergies These days, everybody has one, don't they? Unfortunately, they're more fashionable than a Gucci handbag, but the subject is far more complex than the latest magazine article may have you believe. It's important not to self-prescribe in this area. Here Michelle explains the difference between food allergies and food intolerances or sensitivities, and anaphylactic reactions where the airways swell up so much that the sufferer can have severe breathing problems. This section is very well done, putting the appropriate seriousness on the subject; unfortunately, many people suffer from a hope that they have a food allergy so that they may be given an excuse to avoid certain foods and avoid nourishing themselves properly. Anyone who suspects they have a food allergy really needs to see a doctor for diagnosis.

Excerpts from the Current Inside Story is a round-up of items from the print version of the magazine with many useful web addresses and links for further information. Articles on our recent visit included a piece on diagnosing food allergies and intolerances. They also extend the remit to issues regarding factory farming, BSE, nutrition in general and even allergic dogs.

Excerpts from Our Resource Material has some very useful lists of potentially allergenic ingredients, nutritional services, speciality food suppliers, support groups, and so on.

Booklist is a selection of contemporary titles for sale on the site. In addition, the resources section has an extensive list of relevant books published less recently with useful reviews and publishing information should you wish to track them down.

OTHER FEATURES

Allergy-free recipes, reader feedback, subscription details, and a comprehensive list of links to other food allergy and special diet sites.

An informative site for what can be an extremely serious condition. Inside Story is invaluable for parents and sufferers alike, particularly if food allergies have only been recently diagnosed.

www.macrobiotics.org
Macrobiotics Online

Overall rating: ★ ★ ★			
Classification:	Institute	**Readability:**	★ ★ ★ ★
Updating:	Varies	**Content:**	★ ★ ★ ★
Navigation:	★ ★ ★ ★	**Speed:**	★ ★ ★ ★

US

Produced by the Kushi Institute in America, leading exponents of the macrobiotic philosophy of eating and living, this site is easy to navigate, with the main sections highlighted in a menu panel down the top right of the screen.

SPECIAL FEATURES

Home page features letters and testimonials from people who have cured health problems by converting to a macrobiotic lifestyle. Often these are people previously defined as incurable or inoperable by the medical establishment.

What's new highlights what's new to the site, whether it be new recipes or new products in the online store. On our most recent visit this list showed about three months had gone by with no updates – prior to that there were several.

What is Macrobiotics shows there is no simple definition. Like vegetarianism, macrobiotics is much more than a pattern of healthy eating; it also involves many lifestyle beliefs and choices. They describe the practice as both art and science. Environmental choices are an integral part of it – macrobiotics is not just the choice of grains and particular vegetables for dinner.

Library is a fascinating collection of articles. Illness recovery stories play a major role and specific diseases are listed including bulimia, chronic fatigue, leukaemia, brain tumours, arthritis, and migraines. Also here are frequently asked questions about macrobiotics.

Recipes are essential to every macrobiotic cook because it's almost impossible to get takeaway food. This section is divided into types of dishes and ingredients. Macrobiotic breakfasts include soft rice porridge, mochi waffles, or steamed greens and miso soup, and there is a little explanatory article on why this is the preferred macrobiotic start to the day. There are some great recipes for macrobiotic desserts too such as pumpkin muffins, grape couscous cake, and even puddings made with parsnips (a traditional sweetener before sugar was invented, by the way).

OTHER FEATURES

Information on the Kushi Institute and its courses, an online store, and links to a variety of organisations and individuals, including British macrobiotic sites.

Macrobiotics is nothing new, but is increasingly being taken seriously as a pattern of eating that can be effective in curing disease. The people behind this site are the world's leading exponents of the macrobiotic lifestyle, so this is a key point of reference.

www.nourishnet.com
Nourish Net

Overall rating: ★ ★ ★			
Classification:	Ezine	Readability:	★ ★ ★ ★
Updating:	Monthly	Content:	★ ★ ★ ★
Navigation:	★ ★ ★ ★	Speed:	★ ★ ★ ★

US

Nourish Net was set up by web design professionals Ekistics with a view to creating a community of people interested in weight management and how healthy weight can be achieved. The site offers a variety of free services and information for dieters with the option to become a member and pay for further services such as weigh-ins. 'It's easy to get started', they say on the homepage, and suggest two first steps: keeping a daily log tracking the food you eat, and exercising five days a week. Click on these sections, which are highlighted at the centre of the page, or head to the left-hand menu panel.

SPECIAL FEATURES

Ask Annie answers pleas of help from visitors and comments on issues raised. This sometimes moves into discussion of issues such as depression and isolation, or suffering abuse because of one's size, and so on.

Food Feature is likely to be a recipe from a favourite cookbook, such as the Moosewood Restaurant Low-fat Favourites.

Discoveries recommends the host's favourite new products. These are not strictly relevant to UK consumers, but you may find some good ideas here and be able to buy a similar substitute product. A recent visit found them revealing that Bisquick's reduced fat strawberry shortcake recipe would

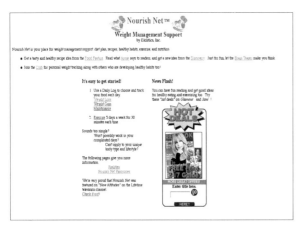

Although this is an ezine, it is in many ways more like an enthusiast's site. It would benefit from more input from well-known nutrition professionals, but there does seem to be a good club atmosphere.

work just as well without the inclusion of butter and could be enhanced by serving with fresh berries.

Brain Teaser is a fun means of helping visitors understand the practicalities of healthy eating. For example, you may be given a typical day's eating log and have to figure out how healthy it really is.

Weight Plan is the largest section and has all the basic information required on achieving healthy weight, whether you want to lose or gain. There are tools, advice on cooking, shopping and eating out, how to assess portion sizes, and so on.

Club One of the main reasons Nourish Net offers a paid-for club with services is that – like every other site – it needs to cover costs and preferably make money. There are a limited number of ways to do this and they have admirably decided that they would rather not travel down the advertising route. But even if you do not want to join and pay a fee, they generously provide a great deal of free information.

www.vegansociety.com
The Vegan Society

Overall rating: ★ ★ ★			
Classification: Society		Readability:	★★★★
Updating:	Varies	Reliability:	★★★★
Navigation:	★★★★	Speed:	★★★★
UK			

This is primarily a philosophical and practical site rather than a destination for vegan cooks. The emphasis is on reasons to be vegan, how to shop vegan and support your local vegan shop, and so on. Those with small screens will need to scroll down to the grid of icons arranged on the centre of the main page. Click on the one that takes your interest or scroll down further to What's New on This Site or the keyword search.

SPECIAL FEATURES

What's New shows the most recent additions to the site, which at the time of our last visit was being updated around weekly, particularly with new links.

Why Vegan? looks in turn at the five main reasons for becoming vegan – animal rights, health or environment issues, use of world resources, and spiritual beliefs. 'All the health benefits of the vegetarian diet come from its vegan component', they argue, pointing out that while meat has 40 per cent calories from fat, cheese has around 70 per cent. They bring in results of recent research to further the points raised. The idea is that, having read this section, vegans will be well-armed to cope with any aggressive questioning about the vegan lifestyle choice whether from relatives, friends and associates, or the media.

News includes recent press releases about Vegan Society

activities plus the organisation's comment on current issues. All are archived and dated. Important too, are the updates to the Vegan Society's key publications, Animal Free Shopper and Vegan Travel Guide.

Information sheets are offered on aspects of vegan nutrition, health and lifestyle such as calcium, protein, how to lose weight on a vegan diet, how to be a gluten-free vegan, making soya milk and tofu, vegan pregnancies, and issues regarding materials such as silk, wool, leather, humane pest control, and so on. There are some recipes are to be found in this section, such as a variety of vegan cakes.

Vegan products is a list of companies and products allowed to carry the Vegan Society trademark.

OTHER FEATURES

Sales of Vegan Society books and other merchandise, local society contact details, membership information, and lots of links listed under International Vegan organisations. These

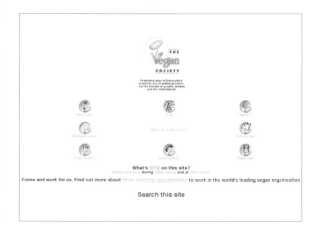

include Beauty without Cruelty (India), Vegan Bikers, and Garden O'Vegan, a vegan farming commune in Hawaii.

An interesting site for the would-be vegan, with several persuasive arguments. However, more could be done to support vegans by providing interactive facilities such as forums, discussion boards, and so on, to create a better sense of community. Also, if you're a vegan looking for culinary inspiration, you won't find much here – head to The Vegan Chef (see p. 89) instead.

OTHER SITES OF INTEREST

5 a Day Campaign
www.5aday.com
This site from the Produce for Better Health Foundation aims to help Americans increase their fruit and vegetable consumption to an average of five or more portions a day. Charts show an impressive increase in awareness since the campaign started. It's a well-designed site, with nutritionally analysed recipes, and plenty of good tips on sneaking fruit and veg into your diet and ways to make veg appealing to kids.

All Recipes
www.allrecipes.com
This general recipe site boasts around 1500 recipes in its special diets section divided into diabetic, vegetarian and vegan, egg-free, gluten-free, and sugar-free. You can save them all to your personal recipe box. This site has a lovely design and it's much easier to use and better edited than

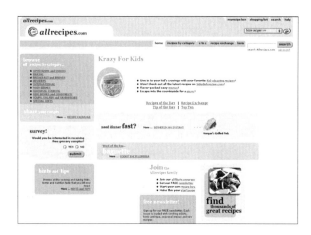

many of the larger recipe collections online. You can interact with other visitors and contribute and rate recipes yourself.

Fatfree: The Low Fat Vegetarian Recipe Archive
www.fatfree.com
The Low Fat Vegetarian Recipe Archive contains well over 4000 recipes plus a link to the USDA nutrient database. You can submit your own recipes. There are around 50 searchable categories including breakfast, pizzas, casseroles, polenta, and stuffed vegetables. Or you can check out the regional selections such as Indian, Mexican, Japanese, or recipes related to specific foods such as seitan, tofu, and beans. Dishes are trawled from other areas of the web and collected from magazines, but there are some great ideas. UK visitors may have to make substitutions for ready-made products not available in Britain, but this site is worth a visit, particularly for vegan cooks.

Healthy Weight Network
www.healthyweightnetwork.com
This is the website of a brilliant American journal which aims to supply interested people with authoritative information about weight and weight management. It's serious, informative, and an excellent source of guidance if you are keen to break a pattern of yo-yo dieting. The dieting industry tends to get a bit of stick, but there are some programmes they are prepared to recommend and you can buy books on them from the site.

Overeaters Anonymous
www.overeatersanonymous.org
Although it's a huge international organisation, Overeaters Anonymous is staunchly uncommercial. This site explains the philosophy on which the non-profit group is based and its programme. Handy too is the description of a typical member, so it's possible to get an inkling of whether or not it's for you, but the only requirement is a commitment to try and stop compulsive overeating.

Shape Up America!
www.shapeup.org
Shape Up America! is an excellent site from a highly reputable group including Dr Koop (see p. 43). The Cyber Kitchen facility, while a little slow to use, is a handy resource for healthy meal planning and dietary analysis. The site also emphasises the importance of increasing activity levels for health benefits.

Symply Too Good To Be True
www.symplytoogood.com.au
'All your favourite recipes! Now guilt free...' is the headline on this Australian site owned by Annette Sym, who has made a successful career of recipe makeovers and lowering the fat content of traditional dishes. The site aims to promote her books, but some recipes are supplied free and you can see it works – Annette bravely provides before and after shots of herself in a swimsuit.

The Fruitarian Foundation
www.fruitarian.com

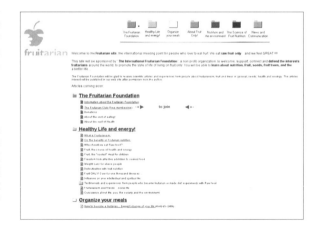

Although it is not well-maintained or updated, this is a good information site for anyone interested in pursuing a fruitarian lifestyle. It explains the basics of the philosophy, how to make the transition to such a diet and provides some insight into the need for support from other fruitarians. In terms of regular community interaction however, you are likely to find the Living and Raw Foods (see p. 88) site more active.

The Healthy Fridge
www.healthyfridge.org
'Open the door to a healthy heart' at this site which offers practical tips for a heart-healthy fridge. Ideas we liked included going over your fridge once a month to throw out the less healthy foods, hiding desserts so that you can forget about them, dividing your fridge up like the healthy eating food pyramid so that you can easily see the more-often and less-often foods, and freezing fruit to eat as snacks. The FAQ section covers subjects such as whether to buy butter or margarine, or how to shop quickly so that you're not so busy that you resort to takeaways. You can post questions too, or peruse some of the fine articles on nutrition.

Chapter 5

exercise

This is not the shopping chapter. You do not need to pay an online personal trainer a subscription fee to send weekly emails telling you to hit the gym, accompanied as they usually are with advertisements promoting huge discounts on bottles of weight loss tablets. For starters, loads of sites will do that for you for free. Second, free or not, it's just a mental prompt. Online personal training is, by its very nature, not personal at all. An email cannot stand next to you at the weight machine urging you to complete another five reps. Of course, it seems cheaper than one-to-one real life training – it has to be, because it's ineffective and poor value for money.

But that does not mean the internet is not a good source of motivation and support when it comes to exercising. There are many magazine-style sites, with articles written by experts, suggested workout plans, illustrated instructions for performing exercises, and advice on how to achieve a balance of fitness. You can find a health club in your area and perhaps meet a workout buddy, either someone who lives nearby or on the other side of the world, through a message board or in a chat room.

A word of warning about community facilities on health sites: it's all very well to share experiences and information but the opinion of a regular person posted on a message board is not the same as the advice of an experienced professional, no matter how authoritative what they say may appear to you. Furthermore, some message boards are badly monitored and controlled (there is a tradition on the internet of non-censorship) and some unscrupulous businesses try to sell their products by 'recommending' them as part of a posted message. You wouldn't give these people the time of day if they approached you on the high street; don't do it on the internet.

Remember that your ultimate aim in learning about exercise is to actually do it. Surfing fitness sites is not the same as participating in exercise and sports, although it can make you feel virtuous. The more you sit at a computer, the more sedentary you are. If you work in an office all day, the last thing you should be doing in your leisure time is surfing (sans board and waves) for hours. Get out and get active.

www.efit.com
eFit: The Online Health and Fitness Network

Overall rating: ★ ★ ★ ★ ★			
Classification:	Ezine	Readability:	★ ★ ★ ★ ★
Updating:	Daily	Reliability:	★ ★ ★ ★ ★
Navigation:	★ ★ ★ ★ ★	Speed:	★ ★ ★ ★ ★

US

The homepage of this lively and authoritative site is large and diverse. You can choose from the simple menu strip across the top of the page, the subject-specific channels in the panel down the left, the keyword search facility, or one of the daily highlighted features. First-timers and those new to fitness should go first to the basics section. To access some sections, it's necessary to take out free membership to the site.

SPECIAL FEATURES

Basics is divided into subject categories along the lines of the site channels – cardio fitness, cooking & nutrition, cycling, and so on. This is the place to come for a thorough grounding in the activities you are looking to incorporate into your lifestyle. Within each subject area there is a series of short articles: Tennis Basics, for example, includes the most frequently asked questions about tennis, what gear to wear, how to warm up, how to get the most out of lessons, what to expect from different courts, playing doubles, playing singles, nutrition for tennis players, common injuries, and more, including a link to the article 'Five beginner's fitness mistakes to avoid'. It's a well-written, comprehensive, and informative section, larger in itself than many other health websites.

Morphover is an interesting service that aims to help you visualise yourself with a healthier, trimmer figure. The premise is that studies increasingly recognise positive visualisation as a key to weight loss success. You send eFit a digital picture of yourself in jpg format, they 'morph' it for you and return a picture of yourself 15lb lighter to stick on your fridge.

News features daily stories from media bureaus such as HealthSCOUT and Associated Press. They could be a response to the latest health research findings, the launch of a new nutrition campaign, reports of a herbal remedy causing damage to the body, or similar.

Cardio Fitness covers indoors and out, home-based and gym. Learn how to get the most from a stairclimber (a tremendous number of people use this machine incorrectly), new fitness moves to help improve your sport, or injury prevention.

Cooking & Nutrition provides recipes, inspirational articles on healthy ingredients, and responds to health discoveries and studies. Typical recipes include Arizona chilli, broccoli and chicken casserole, and banana pie, and there are features on the benefits of eating seasonal fruits and vegetables, how to substitute low-fat products for high-fat ingredients in recipes, and comment on the latest report that eating eggs everyday is perfectly okay for healthy people.

Cycling offers plenty of advice on the nuts and bolts of being a cyclist, such as how to adjust your bike to relieve aches and pains, when to replace your helmet, and how to tell if you need new tyres. Columnist Edmund R. Burke, PhD, provides instruction on bike skills for a more efficient and safer ride.

Diet & Weight Loss analyses the latest diet books on the market and doesn't pull any punches with its criticism so you know which tempting titles to avoid. Also here are inspiring success stories of people who have lost large amounts of weight through the American non-profit organisation Take Off Pounds Sensibly (known as TOPS).

Fit Style includes recommendations of the latest gadgets and accessories for fitness enthusiasts, plus a Spa of the Week review. Our most recent visit saw reviewers recommending low-tech items such as a new skipping rope, collapsible water bottles for riding and hiking, and the new fitness shoe, jump boots, which turn you into a walking trampoline – and are apparently brilliant.

Golf It's more than a stroll round the course with occasional stops to swing a stick, as eFit demonstrates in this channel for those ready to take their golf games to a new level. There are exercises and workout programmes here specially designed to improve your swing speed, driving power, or ability to get round the course, and articles on the finer points of technique, such as theories of club grip.

Healthy Living has a broad remit. Articles on a recent visit ranged from why heartburn should be taken seriously and how vitamin E may cut the risk of stroke, to DIY physical therapy and injury treatment, and choosing the best chair for your office.

Kids' Health is written for parents rather than children and covers subjects such as puberty blues and going to camp.

Men's Health covers aspects of popular psychology as well as nutrition for men, and inspiring tales of men in the health professions. Also here is a regular diary column from an eFit editor struggling to become as fit and active as his job title suggests.

Olympic Sports The primary focus here is American sports stars, but this is an interesting channel where the male and female athletes reveal their programmes for recovery from injuries and how they prepare physically and mentally for competition.

Running covers aspects of training such as why a good hill section could benefit your training program, the pros and cons of treadmills and outdoor running, how to run at night if you can't fit it in during the day, plus features on running celebrities such as victorious marathoners.

Seniors' Health suggests ways in which staying active during later years can maintain happiness, why the old-fashioned callisthenics you're used to is still good for fitness, how to start a fitness programme in later years, or why making a special effort to eat fish could help prevent deterioration of eyesight.

Strength Training includes articles on aspects of technique, such as how changing the grip you use can work different muscles, designing your workout programme (why squats won't make your backside big), or nutrition for building strength.

Swimming Beginners and less confident swimmers are given plenty of support here but there's also insight into how exciting and technical the sport can become – there are articles here on new swimming strokes, and equipment that can help you train and perform better.

Yoga & Mind-Body Even ancient fitness regimes such as yoga and t'ai chi experience innovations, and this is the place to find out about them. Typical articles include how a chi ball can enhance your exercise routine, how to remain Zen-like at work, simple yoga poses, and quick morning workouts.

OTHER FEATURES

There are loads of other sections, including Snow Sports, Teens' Health, Tennis, Sports Medicine, Walking & Hiking, Women's Health, free diet and exercise programmes, healthy restaurant locator (US only), gym locator (US only), eFitTV, and a health and medical dictionary.

eFit is a particularly good choice if you are thinking of taking up a sport or activity, but also has many enjoyable magazine-style features for leisurely reading.

---

www.primusweb.com/fitnesspartner
The Fitness Jumpsite

Overall rating: ★ ★ ★ ★ ★			
Classification:	Homepage	Readability:	★ ★ ★ ★ ★
Updating:	Frequently	Reliability:	★ ★ ★ ★ ★
Navigation:	★ ★ ★ ★ ★	Speed:	★ ★ ★ ★ ★

US

Your connection to a lifestyle of fitness, nutrition and health' is the slogan under the banner, but this site is more than a launch pad to other sites and articles. It provides tools and support for fitness enthusiasts and a library of expert articles. The stylish homepage is extremely easy to navigate – the tools are at the top, the library down the bottom; simply click on the section you want. Right down the bottom of the screen – keep scrolling – is a keyword search facility.

SPECIAL FEATURES

Getting and Staying Active New additions to these archives are highlighted, and on our recent visit, the latest article was one offering safety tips for cardio kick boxing classes, which have seen a recent surge in popularity. Other typical subjects include why having a dog can help you stick to a fitness regime, what to do when you realise your workout has become stale, and how to work exercise into your busy day. Some of these features come from exercise bodies such as IDEA, the leading international health and fitness industry membership organisation. Others are written by noted personal trainers and exercise specialists.

Nutrition Made Easy Are you taking vitamin supplements for the right reasons? How can you follow the principles of good nutrition when you are on the go? Do you realise that stress could be helping to make you fat? These are typical features in this large, informative section.

Managing Your Weight is not about feeling deprived, according to the Fitness Jumpsite. Here you will find many strategies for success, practical and psychological tips, advice on how to overcome weight loss plateaus, prevent the development of eating disorders in children, and include cookies in a healthy eating plan.

Fitness Equipment offers plenty of advice on buying fitness equipment and accessories with comparative trials and articles on subjects such as the 'ten common equipment-buying mistakes'.

Lifestyle Focus Mind-body and beauty issues are covered here along with subjects such as tanning, smoking, and diabetes.

Book Reviews Knowledge is a powerful tool, as this site often states, and this section features short reviews of several specialist books on the market. You won't find gimmicky diets and theories here, but sound, proven advice from publishers of the industry's more serious titles.

Activity Calorie Calculator Click on this if you would like to analyse the number of calories burnt performing particular activities – there are 158 to choose from. Unlike charts that generalise how many calories are burned while participating in exercise and sports, this calculator bases the information on your weight, so is a little more accurate.

Fitness Forum encourages you to find a fitness partner or email pal. This section is well attended, mainly by American women of various ages. The founders of this site first met on an internet fitness discussion group, so well understand its value. The bulletin boards are also well attended, with most participants being very knowledgeable amateurs. Also here is an invitation to share thoughts about what fitness means to you.

OTHER FEATURES

Trophy Case features media accolades won by the site, and there's the opportunity to buy and sell fitness equipment.

With its clear, simple design and authoritative features, this upbeat site is definitely one to bookmark if you want to start leading an active life or make fitness buddies.

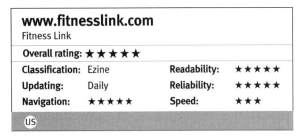

www.fitnesslink.com
Fitness Link

Overall rating: ★ ★ ★ ★ ★			
Classification: Ezine		**Readability:**	★ ★ ★ ★ ★
Updating: Daily		**Reliability:**	★ ★ ★ ★ ★
Navigation: ★ ★ ★ ★ ★		**Speed:**	★ ★ ★

US

'Reshape your world' at this authoritative, cutting-edge site full of fitness information delivered with a sense of humour. Unfortunately, it's slow to load, but the menu panel does eventually appear down the left-hand side of the page. Alternatively, you can scroll down beneath that to do a keyword search, or simply click on one of the features highlighted at the centre of the homepage.

SPECIAL FEATURES

Athletic Adventures covers outdoor adventure sports, sports fitness, and fitness travel. Typical articles might cover death-defying BASE jumping (BASE stands for buildings, antennas, spans, and earth), power golfing, how to get more out of tandem cycling, plans to open fitness centres in airports, or what to do if the airport you're passing through still doesn't have a gym. Previous articles are archived and, at the base of each, there are links to related features.

Exercise Encyclopedia 'Learn to Burn' with this library of photo and video demonstrations accompanied by a glossary defining all the basic fitness terms. There are also features on whether or not there is a best time to exercise, tracking exercise performance, beginners' guides to strength training and body building, specific workout programmes, and the latest cardio workouts. Pieces on issues such as treadmill versus outdoor running are backed up by the latest expert input and research.

Virtual Gym is the place to go if you've ever found yourself standing bewildered in a gym and unable to get the attention of the instructor. Here former Mr Universe bodybuilding champion Doug Brignole explains the use of dozens of pieces of gym equipment and machines. Scroll down to click on the individual coloured muscles on the anatomical drawings – this will take you to a picture of the equipment, then to a description of the exercise, its benefits and uses, and good tips on how to perform to the best advantage.

Home Gym is quite different from the virtual gym – it is a collection of articles on how to work out at home, backed by advice on purchasing fitness equipment and videos for home use and a series of workout routines (plus advice on how to devise your own). The site alerts users to the cons of the trade, the weird and not-wonderful pieces of exercise equipment advertised on cable TV and in the classified sections of magazines. On abdominal devices they say: 'Save your bucks!'

Nutrition & Diet Weight loss and dieting, healthy eating, recipes, supplements and herbs, and sports nutrition are all featured in this informative and diverse channel. Discover the keys to healthy weight loss and maintenance, find which supplements are best for body builders or how to slim down just before a competition, which oils you should use for cooking, and whether a glass of beer could actually do you some good. Previous articles are archived and contributors include respected authors and journalists in the field.

Mind & Body Use your brain to help you get a stronger, fitter body – a 'weak mind will equal a weak body', according to one of the expert contributors, John Abdo, a consultant and professor of fitness training. This excellent section covers current as well as future trends in its Mindful Workouts session. Here you can find out what your first Pilates session may be like, or get the low-down on Chin Na, a system of self-defence for people who are not particularly strong. The motivation section features articles such as 'Commit to Get Fit' and what to do when 'It's Mind Over Matter – and Your Body's the Matter!'. Scroll down for Stress Management, another key section, with features on techniques such as visualisation, progressive relaxation, and meditation.

Men's Locker Room The testosterone oozes from the screen in this macho channel complete with a full-colour, full-muscled fitness model pin-up of the week. Do you feel like a prat in aerobics classes or the weight room? There are guys' guides to looking cool in both the Sports and Fitness sections. Also here, a section called Strength, Supplements and Sex for the body building fraternity. 'Men – train with a lady for better results' and 'A Different Abdominal Exercise ...Really!' are typical stories.

Women's Locker Room Girls get a pin-up of the week, too, but on our last visit, the floppy haired, doe-eyed chap looked as though he wouldn't last five seconds arm-wrestling the woman posing in the Men's Locker Room. More serious stuff in this channel includes features such as the prevalence of iron deficiency in active women, how to get a whole family active, and how to exercise safely during pregnancy. Popular American fitness guru Denise Austin answers questions from visitors – you need to click on the 'Ask a Question' link in order to read other people's questions (this will take you through to www.deniseaustin.com, but you still have access to the www.fitnesslink.com menu). This section is broken down into subject areas such as weight loss, aches and pains, equipment and apparel, pregnancy, and trouble spots, as well as general fitness questions.

Pro's Center may be of interest to sport and exercise enthusiasts as well as professionals, as there are articles here on famous fitness heroes such as Olympic gold medallist Jackie Joyner-Kersee and how to become a fitness instructor, as well as features such as 'Keeping older exercisers in your fitness class' and 'Promoting your fitness business'.

Total Wellness 'Live Long and Prosper' is the subtitle of this channel, added to the site comparatively recently. Not many articles are in place yet, although typical subjects are fitness for kids, anti-ageing ideas, and fitness for the over-fifties, plus features on integrative medicine treatments, such as aromatherapy.

The Juice Bar is the interactive section of the site. In addition to the 'find a friend in fitness' scheme, forums and discussion groups, and competitions, there is a regular cartoon, and tools to calculate your fitness level by analysing your body mass index and target heart rate, and a facility to log your workouts.

OTHER FEATURES

Today's News, Your Daily Dose, newsletter, and many links within the articles to sites by featured fitness professionals and services. There is also a large dedicated links section with sites assessed and rated – choose the type of site you are looking for from the pull-down menu.

This is an excellent link to a more active life.

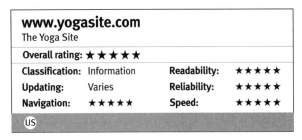

www.yogasite.com
The Yoga Site

Overall rating: ★ ★ ★ ★ ★			
Classification:	Information	**Readability:**	★ ★ ★ ★ ★
Updating:	Varies	**Reliability:**	★ ★ ★ ★ ★
Navigation:	★ ★ ★ ★ ★	**Speed:**	★ ★ ★ ★ ★

US

'An eclectic collection of yoga connections' is promised by this attractive American site. The layout is simple, with the main sections set in buttons down the left of the screen. You can go directly to the new additions by clicking on the highlighted links in the centre of the page. Scroll beneath these to find a list of other recent features, which will take you direct to some fine articles.

SPECIAL FEATURES

Yoga Postures A selection of basic postures is given here with descriptions of how to perform them in text and cartoons. It's a long list, requiring a lot of scrolling, unless the particular posture you want to view is listed at the side, in which case you can click on the name and jump to it. The cute stick-figure drawings are hardly detailed, but make each posture seem achievable, even if you know they're tough.

Yoga Retreats While most of those featured are in the USA and Canada, this is a somewhat international list featuring retreats in countries as diverse as Spain, France, Peru, Mexico, Costa Rica, and the Bahamas. Some centres are reviewed, making this a fine holiday guide for the yoga enthusiast.

Yoga Styles The three main styles – Ashtanga, Iyengar, and Viniyoga – are all derived from the teachings of Krishnamacharya, a famous teacher at the yoga institute of the Mysore Palace in India. However, there are differences which lead to some people feeling more comfortable with one style than another. This section explains the differences between them and other styles of yoga, including Bikram, Sivananda, Integral, and Anusara.

Questions and Answers New queries are highlighted in this section which considers problems from amateurs as well as those interested in becoming yoga teachers. If you've ever wondered what 'Om' means, how many times a week you should practise yoga, or whether it will make you taller or cure varicose veins, this is the place to come. You can also submit questions.

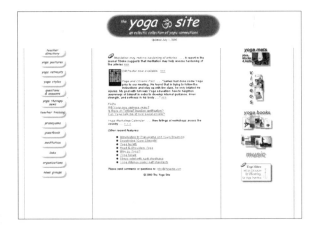

Yoga Therapy News 'Discover what science is learning about yoga' is the way they wryly put it. This is an interesting series of articles on subjects such as yoga for MS, asthma and carpal tunnel syndrome, some with specific exercise recommendations. Stories are archived for reference.

Pranayama offers information on yogic breathing techniques such as nadi shodhana, or the sweet breath, which is a method of breathing using alternate nostrils.

Meditation is a basic guide to the subject from a yoga perspective, in which it is considered the highest practice and the final step before bliss, whereas other traditions seek 'merely' intense awareness. A few meditation exercises are given here to get you started.

OTHER FEATURES

Teacher directory, teacher training, guest book, yoga organisations, recommended news groups, and shopping. Plenty of links are given to relevant articles, magazines, mailing lists, news groups, and so on, both in the dedicated links section and within relevant articles on the site.

Clear, well-written, beautifully designed, informative, authoritative...if only the yoga itself were this easy and enjoyable.

www.acefitnesslink.org

American Council on Exercise

Overall rating: ★ ★ ★ ★

Classification:	Ezine	**Readability:**	★ ★ ★ ★ ★
Updating:	Daily	**Reliability:**	★ ★ ★ ★ ★
Navigation:	★ ★ ★ ★ ★	**Speed:**	★ ★ ★ ★

US

The Amercian Council on Exercise is a non-profit organisation promoting active lifestyles and their positive effects, as well as protecting the public against unsafe and ineffective fitness products and trends. The centre of the homepage highlights new additions to the site. The menu panel down the left of the screen offers buttons for various departments, much of which is relevant only to Americans (such as how to find an ACE-certified trainer, or become one). Another menu panel on the right explains a little more about what may be found in the departments.

SPECIAL FEATURES

What's Hot could be an excerpt from a new book certified or recommended by ACE, but is always much more than just a few paragraphs – a real flavour of the title is given, making it very tempting.

ACE Fit Facts covers more than 80 health-and-fitness related subjects, which incorporate nutrition and medical health matters as well as activity.

ACE Store includes not just books but study materials and manuals. Committed exercisers and professionals may find some good products not widely available elsewhere. Also here is a range of free products from ACE, such as the Health E-tips Newsletter for exercise enthusiasts, and Pro Tips Online for fitness professionals. Products may be purchased in bulk.

ACE Fitness Matters offers subscriptions to the magazine of the same name, a powerful exercise industry watchdog lauded by the Wall Street Journal. Its reports have resulted in dubious product infomercials being removed from the airwaves and have saved consumers millions of dollars each year.

Fact of the Day is an item aiming to destroy myths surrounding exercise and fitness, for example, 'exercises such as crunches or leg lifts improve the tone and endurance of muscles, but they don't burn fat'.

OTHER FEATURES

About ACE, Find an ACE Pro, ACE Store, Press Center, ACE Faculty, and more.

An essential site of reference for fitness professionals and anyone with a serious interest in exercise, but ACE is also an authoritative resource for non-experts and beginners, as it is free of fads and junk science.

www.justmove.org
The American Heart Association Fitness Center

Overall rating: ★ ★ ★			
Classification:	Campaign	Readability:	★ ★ ★ ★ ★
Updating:	Varies	Reliability:	★ ★ ★ ★
Navigation:	★ ★ ★ ★ ★	Speed:	★ ★ ★ ★ ★

US

Fighting heart disease and stroke are the primary concerns of the American Heart Association (AHA), and this site is dedicated to promoting the role of fitness in these efforts. Once you have entered the site, the homepage is very easy to understand, with the main features listed down the left-hand side of the screen. The Bayer corporation is a sponsor of this site and so there is much information peppered throughout the site on aspirin.

SPECIAL FEATURES

Exercise Diary is a free tool that allows you to track your progress online – daily, weekly or monthly – and receive feedback reports and statistical summaries. You can also sign up for a virtual personal trainer, who will send you encouragement and suggestions to help you stick to your plan. Parts of the site were experiencing technical difficulties at the time of our reviews; however, the AHA promised to notify anyone who typed in their email address when the tools were back online.

Fitness News encompasses the latest health, heart, and fitness information from around the world, including reports from the British media. The daily news is supplied by Reuters and previous stories are archived. There is also an FAQ section particularly useful for people who have been sedentary for some time, and a list of health facts relating to cardiovascular disease (still America's biggest killer), exercise for various age groups and abilities, obesity, sex, and much, much more. Where appropriate, these information pages contain handy tools and charts to help you plan and track your personal health campaign.

My Fitness asks what fitness category (low active, active, or special care) you fall into and offers advice from the fact sheets – peruse the list of titles and choose which you want to read. We felt this section was a little too simple when it came to classifying levels of activity.

Measure Up compares your details to those of the American population, using the AHA's national fitness database.

Cyber Teams is the forum section that provides a medium for those with fitness-related interests to connect with each other. The site offers several subject areas including how to stay motivated, nutrition, and sports.

OTHER FEATURES

US events section, search facility, site map, and many choices of e-cards.

The AHA site may appeal more to people in their middle and late years – it's well designed and has lots of good information, but does not try to be funky.

www.fun-and-fitness.com			
Fun and Fitness			
Overall rating: ★ ★ ★ ★			
Classification:	Ezine	Readability:	★ ★ ★ ★
Updating:	Varies	Reliability:	★ ★ ★ ★
Navigation:	★ ★ ★ ★	Speed:	★ ★ ★ ★
UK			

Andrew Wright is a fitness instructor based in Essex who has designed this site with the aim of being informative but simple – for more in-depth information he recommends you head to the book section. The slogan is 'Get fit, stay fit and enjoy it!' The weight-lifter cartoon on the front page suggests this site is designed to appeal to men who are already quite into fitness, though this is not really the case. Enter the site, then choose the category in which you are interested from the list of buttons at the left of the screen. These buttons change as you enter each section, and you'll find it easiest to keep using them to navigate rather than scroll to the bottom of the screen.

SPECIAL FEATURES

Information Zone includes tips on training, aerobic, and anaerobic fitness, surviving exercise classes, and how to exercise in hot weather. Many tips are given, and they are well written and to the point.

Muscle Zone is divided into muscle groups, such as abdominals, shoulder muscles, lower back, legs, and so on. The technical names, descriptions, and main actions of the muscle are given. Scroll down to beneath the anatomical drawings to find which exercises are recommended for each muscle.

Nutrition Zone is a detailed section with food types, energy systems, body composition, weight control, and the relationship between nutrition and exercise covered. The advice here is based on sound accepted theory rather than fads or gimmicks. The energy systems section is quite technical, but uses diagrams to illustrate the theories.

Fitness Bookshelf recommends several titles including general fitness, muscle, and nutrition books. The recommendations are annotated by Fun and Fitness with the books available for sale through Amazon.

Fun Zone includes fitness e-cards, polls, chat, and forum sessions plus fitness hangman – which is way too easy.

Fitness Focus was a recent addition to the site at the time of our last review. It seeks to recommend clubs, associations and organisations that promote a healthy and fit lifestyle. The British Rope Skipping Association was one featured, and site visitors were invited to send in their suggestions.

OTHER FEATURES

Feedback, questions, and book sales. There are also several links to other fitness sites, magazines, companies and organisations, with Andrew Wright's favourites recommended on a dedicated page. You can search the links section by subject category.

Although the tone and design suggest at times that this is an enthusiast's homepage, the text comes from an authoritative professional. We found good tips here we'd never read before.

www.turnstep.com
Turnstep

Overall rating: ★ ★ ★ ★			
Classification:	Information	Readability:	★ ★ ★ ★
Updating:	Varies	Reliability:	★ ★ ★ ★
Navigation:	★ ★ ★ ★	Speed:	★ ★ ★ ★

US

A glance through the results of the site polls shows that most visitors to Turnstep are fitness teachers, but exercise enthusiasts looking for new ways to add spice to their at-home workouts will love this site too. Its primary purpose is to catalogue aerobic dance steps and patterns and, on our last visit, the site offered 7,243, but the figure is increasing all the time. The design is basic and functional, and relatively easy to navigate. The main proportion of the homepage is devoted to cataloguing the latest steps. First-time visitors should scroll to the link at the bottom left of the screen headed About the Pictures.

SPECIAL FEATURES

About the Pictures is the key to understanding the animated step descriptions. As the drawings explain point by point, the red shoe is the right foot, the yellow shoe is the left foot, and so on. Step fans will be able to look at the animations and pick up most steps quickly because the format is admirably intuitive, however anyone more than a little uncoordinated will appreciate the simple explanations.

Turnstep News contains details of recent additions to the site and reports on any fixed errors. Earlier this year, people from Guyana, Chile, and Jamaica added steps to the site, bringing the number of contributing countries to 63.

Latest Moves are given in animated pictures and are very easy to follow. Clicking on More Moves underneath the featured steps will take you through to the Aerobics Dictionary, which contains all the most popular dance steps in animated form, from the A-step to the V-, X-, Y-, and Z-steps, via the mambo, cha-cha-cha, flamingo, and helicopter.

Latest 50 Patterns As this section demonstrates, it's not all about aerobic dance and step. Also here are moves for cardio boxing workouts, body sculpting, cycling, and aquatic workouts. People with really fancy footwork can attempt Double Step sequences, using two step benches at once. Some of the more advanced steps are written in jargon and do not have pictures so can be difficult to follow. The pull-down menus at the base of this section allow you to search the site by type of exercise (funk, warm-up, abs, slide, and so on) or by month. Beneath that is a link to the statistics behind the various patterns – there are more than 4,200 for step classes, nearly 400 for box aerobics, and so on.

Adaptive Aerobics offers advice for professionals on how they can make their classes more inclusive and integrate all abilities and disabilities.

Aerobics FAQ can also be read in html or downloaded as a text-heavy version. It answers basic questions such as 'What is aerobic exercise?', 'How do I determine my target heart rate?', 'How do I know when I'm exercising hard enough to burn fat?', and 'If I do lots of outer thigh exercises will that part of my body slim down first?'.

OTHER FEATURES

Video Reviews, Bulletin Board, Job Board, and links to the site sponsors who offer exercise music for sale.

Home exercisers will love this – there are plenty of ideas for adding spice and fun to dance-style step workouts.

---

www.yoyoga.com
Yo Yoga

Overall rating: ★ ★ ★ ★			
Classification:	Homepage	**Readability:**	★ ★ ★ ★
Updating:	Fortnightly	**Reliability:**	★ ★ ★ ★ ★
Navigation:	★ ★ ★ ★ ★	**Speed:**	★ ★ ★ ★ ★

US

Joan Budilovsky is a yoga teacher and author of the Complete Idiot's Guide to Yoga (plus a book on meditation and another on massage). She is also the host of this charming site which attracts many visitors from Britain, or as she likes to call it, 'Merry ol' England'. The homepage will typically contain atmospheric photographs of natural landscapes and an inspirational quote. Navigate using the series of buttons across the top of the screen.

SPECIAL FEATURES

Asana is the yoga pose of the week, with written instructions for performing it, plus a photograph. Included are visualisation and meditation suggestions.

Philosophy It's important to remember that yoga is a practice of body and mind, says Joan, and in this section she offers explanation and insight into various aspects of the philosophical and spiritual side. 'This is not meant to be a guilt trip exercise,' she says. 'It is meant as an exercise in awareness...My Yo Yoga renditions are meant to encourage you to read and reflect more on this simple thread and how it weaves through your individual life.'

Yoga Tips is a brief but good section, with a different tip featured each fortnight. A typical example answers whether you should meditate or practise your yoga postures if feeling depressed. The answer? Postures, because they help move impurities and negativity out of the body. Joan recommends meditation for those occasions when you're already feeling good.

Yo Joan Readers and fans can send Joan their questions, which she answers effectively using her obvious expertise and sensitivity. Fans of agony aunt columns will like this one.

Recipe One or two vegetarian recipes are supplied by readers each fortnight, with prizes going to the best.

Bookstore features books and audio tapes by Joan.

Yo Yoga is more personal, spiritual, and touchy-feely than The Yoga Site (see p. 108) – but that's part of its charm, and perhaps a reason why some will prefer it. Joan is certainly an excellent advertisement for the practice, and her warmth and kindness in dealing with questions from visitors and fans are quite inspiring.

www.adidas.co.uk/running
Adidas: The Runner

Overall rating: ★ ★ ★			
Classification:	Information	Readability:	★ ★ ★ ★
Updating:	Varies	Reliability:	★ ★ ★
Navigation:	★ ★ ★ ★	Speed:	★ ★ ★

US

A welcome and much-needed alternative to the superficial and gimmicky www.adidas.com site, this runners' home-page has become quite popular with enthusiasts and has received much publicity. The menu panel down the left of the screen highlights the three main channels, but you can access other aspects of the site via the icons on the right of the screen. Registration (free) is encouraged with the offer of a training diary facility.

SPECIAL FEATURES

What's New unsurprisingly highlights latest additions to the site. On our most recent visit, that was post-marathon advice for people who had attempted the London marathon two months earlier. A click here leads through to a section called News and Features which also had articles on running stars, and an insider's perspective on why Kenya seems to be producing the world's greatest runners.

Get in Touch includes the runner's notice board and a club search facility. The site also offers to help running clubs build their own site. Using these facilities requires registration. The Get Noticed discussion area is well attended, but mainly by people posing questions rather than answering them. This section is also accessed by clicking on the Together heading.

Alone is about the individual runner and is divided into sections on diet, lifestyle, and physiotherapy, as well as training programs. Training tips come from Bud Baldaro, running coach for the Great Britain cross country team. Your Diet includes the 'golden rules' of nutrition.

Relay includes a facility to help you find your local running store, advice on buying shoes and running clothes. Amongst the Track and Field features are profiles of Adidas-sponsored athletes, results of recent events and a look at how Adidas is helping to promote running in schools. You can also sign up for a monthly running newsletter from Adidas.

Some of the momentum of this fine site seems to have been lost post-London marathon. The features are good but need to be updated more frequently. The site also needs some technical maintenance as a few of the links weren't working properly as we went to press. However, it would be a shame for Adidas to wind this down, as it's a great service to the running community and helpful to those who would like to take up the sport.

OTHER SITES OF INTEREST

Active for Life
www.active.org.uk
A site from the former Health Education Authority, which has morphed into Health Promotion England and the Health Development Authority. Although a little self-consciously groovy, the information here is excellent for people looking to improve their health and fitness.

Health Club Net
www.health-club.net
You can search for a health club in your area from this database of around 5,000 gyms and leisure centres in the UK including Northern Ireland. The list needs more meticulous updating, though it should provide you with useful contact addresses and phone numbers.

IDEA: The Health and Fitness Source
www.ideafit.com
Look here for the experts' views on exercising, a non-dieting approach to healthy eating, how to find the best mind-body class for you, and why you might like to try a particular sport.

Video Fitness
www.videofitness.com
This site is part of the Fitness Online network and offers a venue for fans of fitness videos, incorporating reviews of the latest releases, a video exchange facility, success stories, industry news, and behind-the-scenes articles.

Women's Sport Foundation
www.wsf.org.uk
The homepage of the British Women's Sport Foundation will provide you with a great starting point for taking up a sport. A tremendous number are covered, including popular activities like badminton and soccer as well as less-well-known sports such as lacrosse.

Chapter 6

shopping

It's easy to think, mistakenly, that the whole point of the internet is to buy things online. There is a lot of talk about the internet shopping revolution – and in the long run it probably is a revolution. But while the possibilities get people excited, at the moment it's little more than trumped-up mail order, and only of benefit if it fits your lifestyle. Certainly there are discounted products to be found online, but before pressing the submit button, you need to consider the real cost and convenience of your purchase.

This is not just a matter of adding the charge for the packaging and postage, which usually lifts the price to around the same as you'd pay on the high street. Consider how and when you are you going to receive your shopping. Small, unbreakable and unperishable purchases slip through the letterbox easily enough, but usually items are too large to do that. If there is no safe place for the delivery company to leave things or a trusted home-bound neighbour with whom parcels can be left, you will probably find it necessary to take time off work in order to stay in and take delivery. Sorting out the day your goods will arrive can in itself involve a lot of time spent emailing and making phone calls. And there's nothing quite like the feeling engendered by agreeing to stay in all day to receive a parcel that doesn't arrive. By the time you're spending precious Saturday mornings driving to a depot in the next county to pick the goods up yourself, you will be struggling to remember why you wanted the products in the first place.

Unbelieveable as it may seem, even home workers have trouble with internet shopping. Delivery companies are increasingly unable to guarantee even a half-day in which they will turn up, making it impossible to pop out for anything, let alone a meeting. And if it's clothes or shoes you've purchased and they don't fit properly, you will need to arrange return of the parcel and go through the whole thing again. Retail therapy? No, but you can always refer to websites in the Healthy Living chapter for stress management techniques.

Where internet shopping scores is the ability to find products relatively easily that you may not have been able to get on the high street. For example, until recently, outside speciality shops in the major cities it was difficult to find miso at all, let alone the fine selection offered by mail at www.clearspring.co.uk, where you can also buy the Indonesian speciality soy food tempeh and organic snow-dried tofu from the mountain regions of Japan. A monthly box of these healthy culinary goodies might even be worth staying in for.

www.boots.co.uk
Boots the Chemist

Overall rating: ★ ★ ★ ★ ★			
Classification:	Ecommerce	Readability:	★ ★ ★ ★
Updating:	Monthly	Content:	★ ★ ★ ★
Navigation:	★ ★ ★ ★ ★	Speed:	★ ★ ★ ★ ★

UK 🔒

'It's about being you,' croons the country's leading chemist, and impressively, it is, as the contents of this truly interactive site can be structured to suit your own preferences. If you register for free membership, you are given a brief questionnaire that asks about your main areas of interest, for example health and fitness, alternative health, stress relief, or mother and baby information. Articles and products covering the areas you have chosen will then be presented to you each time you visit the site.

The homepage offers several points of entry. A menu across the top of the page gives a broad overview, and beneath are panels entitled Reading, and Shopping, that highlight the month's features and tips or special offers and seasonal products. Alternatively, select from the pull-down menu headlined 'How do you feel today?' to which you may respond: 'I have PMT', 'I want a body overhaul', 'I feel fluey', or 'I want to sort out my spots'. You will then be presented with brief articles and suggested products relevant to your choice.

SPECIAL FEATURES

Reading Boots' lively and well-written articles are often written by established journalists in the field and feature comments from professional experts. Particularly good is the diary of a cold, which lets you know what to expect

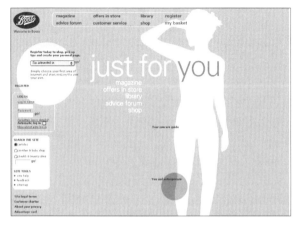

divided into Change Time, Food Time, Outdoor Baby, Baby Indoors, and Before Baby. Click on one of these options and you will be presented with the age ranges of suitable products, which you then choose from to view items. Click again to see enlargements and more product information.

Boots Consultant is an interactive quiz on the subject of complexion that results in recommendations of Boots products for your skin type. They plan to expand this section once its popularity has been established.

OTHER FEATURES

What's New, Index, Customer Services, Help, and Community, which includes not-very-well-attended forums and occasionally the opportunity to ask an expert such as makeup authority Liz Collinge.

The major supermarket food retailers would do well to take a careful look at this site. Although limited in scope by comparison, it works tremendously well, and is interesting, easy, and fun to use.

throughout your relationship with the bug. Other subjects include condoms, sexual equality and responsibility, personal motivation and self-esteem, and how to include healthy fats in the diet, with related articles suggested in the margins. Past and present articles are archived, and you can save your favourite pieces to your personal page. From the articles you can link to related subjects on the forums.

Personal Pages This section lets you store your favourite articles and flags up new promotions available in store relevant to your areas of interest. The calendar facility allows you to set up reminder messages to yourself, and shows public holidays and relevant Boots promotions. You can also view your previous purchases and edit your profile if you decide you would rather see information and products on different subjects.

Shopping is divided into two main categories: health and beauty for women and men, and mother and baby. A variety of brands is offered, not just Boots' own label. Within the health and beauty section is makeup, healthcare such as vitamins and first aid products, the Botanics range, travel and photographic items, and hosiery. Mother and Baby is

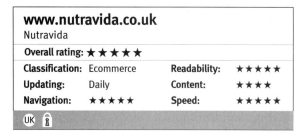

www.nutravida.co.uk
Nutravida

Overall rating: ★ ★ ★ ★ ★			
Classification:	Ecommerce	Readability:	★ ★ ★ ★ ★
Updating:	Daily	Content:	★ ★ ★ ★
Navigation:	★ ★ ★ ★ ★	Speed:	★ ★ ★ ★ ★

UK

Nutravida is the trading name of Oxford Nutraceuticals, a company set up by two businessmen from other areas of the retail trade. The homepage allows you to browse by condition, lifestyle, or type of product, or conduct a keyword/phrase search. Various products, special offers, and ailments are highlighted up front to tempt you.

SPECIAL FEATURES

Aromatherapy is an excellent section with a comprehensive list and useful information, for example, did you know that black pepper essence is incompatible with homeopathic remedies? It is often used in commercial massage blends to relax tired muscles and support healthy respiration but should be avoided if you are pregnant, have high blood pressure or epilepsy. Tisserand supply many of the oils listed here, and others come from Cariad.

Evening Primrose Oil   A quality section with almost too much to choose from. Products are stocked from almost every leading manufacturer, including Solgar, Quest, Seven Seas, and Lamberts. There is also a dry form from Kudos for people who find the beneficial oils difficult to digest.

Slimming   There is a tremendous range of products here, though too much self-prescription is probably foolish. Country Life produces Burn'n'Trim lipotropic amino acids with vitamins and minerals, Diet Power herb and nutrient

formula 'to support appetite control, metabolic efficiency and healthy fat metabolism', and Lipotropic Metabolise to 'support liver and intestinal tract for healthy fat metabolism and levels of fat accumulation with added taurine'. Fat Defense is a 'balanced combination of natural non-stimulating ingredients including tamarind and vital trace minerals', whatever that means...

Green Foods   Another comprehensive selection that includes products based on alfalfa, brewer's yeast, kelp, pollen, royal jelly, spirulina, beetroot, chlorella, lecithin, propolis, and reishi shitake. In some cases, such as chlorella, a choice of brands, sizes and prices is offered.

Special Supplements   Here you'll find shark cartilage, grapefruit seed extract, charcoal, soya isoflavones, co-enzyme Q10 and glucosamine sulphate, amongst others.

Nutravida Packs are ailment-oriented collections that aim to make dietary supplementation simple. Choose from kits such as the menstruation pack, hangover pack, urban living, or executive pressure, with a mixture of products and brands. They rightfully point out that you need to be careful not to exceed recommended dosages and that some packs are unsuitable if pregnant or breastfeeding. There are also beauty-oriented collections such as the new woman home spa kit, with Dead Sea bathing salts, clay face mask, and so on.

OTHER FEATURES

Various products such as flower remedies and digestive aids, books, special offers, contact details, press reports and customer reviews, and a company press pack.

There is a comprehensive selection of both popular and more unusual items. Prices are very competitive, lower than the high street, and include postage and packing in the UK. Delivery is promised within 48 hours and often achieved within 24.

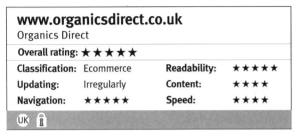

www.organicsdirect.co.uk
Organics Direct

Overall rating: ★ ★ ★ ★			
Classification:	Ecommerce	Readability:	★ ★ ★ ★ ★
Updating:	Irregularly	Content:	★ ★ ★
Navigation:	★ ★ ★ ★ ★	Speed:	★ ★ ★ ★

UK 🔒

Organics Direct is a leading British organic foods home delivery service. In addition to its ecommerce role, the company uses this well illustrated website to promote healthy eating and an anti-GM foods stance. The site loads quite quickly, is easy to move around, and has easy ordering. A useful coding system denotes which products are yeast-free, gluten-free, and wheat-free.

SPECIAL FEATURES

Fields and Orchards is where you'll find the handy fresh vegetable and fruit boxes.

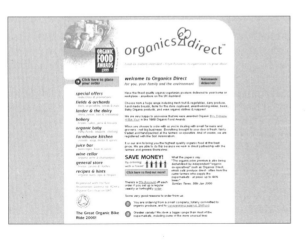

Larder and Dairy includes storecupboard groceries, dairy boxes and an à la carte dairy range. The speciality grains offered include millet, raw buckwheat, barley and quinoa, and there are dried pulses such as adzuki, black turtle, mung and soya beans, and puy lentils. Keen healthy eaters will also be interested in the choice of wholemeal pasta shapes.

Farmhouse Kitchen features some breakfast cereals for special diets such as barley flakes, rice flakes, rye flakes, multigrain flakes, and several mueslis. Here too is textured vegetable protein, available in plain, savoury, and curry flavours.

General Store offers a great selection of books on organic food and juice therapy as well as other health subjects. Organics Direct also sells a large range of juicers including the top-of-the-range, hard-to-get, take-out-a-mortgage Champion models.

Delivery is not as flexible as is perhaps necessary, although you can specify the day of delivery, and for an extra charge, insist that it arrive in the morning. Company addresses are acceptable to Organics Direct, but not to anyone who travels to work by public transport.

OTHER FEATURES

The company sells organic wine and beer, and a few non-food items too. There are inspiring quotes from satisfied customers and media, and links to anti-GM organisations and charities.

A very good site to shop from, provided you can work with their delivery system.

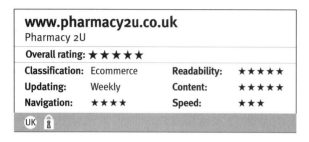

www.pharmacy2u.co.uk
Pharmacy 2U

Overall rating: ★ ★ ★ ★ ★			
Classification:	Ecommerce	**Readability:**	★ ★ ★ ★ ★
Updating:	Weekly	**Content:**	★ ★ ★ ★ ★
Navigation:	★ ★ ★ ★	**Speed:**	★ ★ ★

UK

Pharmacy 2U claims to have been the UK's first online pharmacy and their experience shows in this well-designed and easy-to-use site. Some departments and special offers are highlighted at the centre of the homepage but the key navigational devices are the menu strips across the top and bottom of the screen. For the administrative sections of the site, use the panel down the left-hand side of the screen. You can search the site by brand name using the facility at the top left of the homepage. When clicking through the range of products, you have to use the back buttons a lot, which is rather irritating and slows down the shoping process.

SPECIAL FEATURES

Ask Our Pharmacist is a confidential service offered to individuals with enquiries about health and medication. You can email directly from the link on the homepage, or telephone the freephone helpline.

Private Prescriptions Free UK delivery is offered on private prescriptions. You need to register and log in to use this service.

Medicines Click here and you will be presented with a list of product categories including pain relief, cough, cold and sore throat, skin care and antiseptics, hair and scalp, ear and eye care, oral hygiene, and more. There are 24 products

for sore throat alone, including all major brands listed in alphabetical order. Click on the highlighted name of the product to be taken through to a page offering further product information, including warnings about the circumstances in which the product should not be used and details of its side effects.

Healthcare Parmacy2U has its own label of vitamin and mineral supplements but offers a few major brands, too. This section also contains first aid, foot care, homeopathic remedies, dietary foods and meal replacements, family planning, eye and lens care, and so on.

Personal Care There are 87 shampoos to choose from here, but none of the sexy upmarket celebrity hairdresser shampoos that can be found in supermarkets and Boots these days – a real missed opportunity. Also in this section are everyday dental care products, deodorants, tissues and toilet paper, baby food, bath and shower preparations and so on.

Beauty Fragrance, skin care, suncare and hair colour are available here. There are many esteemed names amongst the perfume list, but only mass-market stuff amongst the skincare.

Disability Aids and Lifestyle Equipment contains a wide variety of items, including a choice of 47 magnotherapy jewellery products, commodes and bedpans, thermometers, anti-allergenic bedding covers, protective bedding and seating, several types of walker, bath seats and bath boards, plus products for aid with eating and drinking. This looks like a very good selection, and a highly convenient way to buy such products.

Best Buys on our most recent visit included a few buy-one-get-one-free offers and one-third off. Delivery is free on all orders over £30 and, for orders of lower value, £2.50 is charged for UK mainland deliveries (a fair rate in our experience).

Links are under the title Health Information and include a selection of UK information sites

OTHER FEATURES

Affiliate programme.

We like this site but think it has little to offer that your local chemist doesn't. It would be enhanced by more speciality and indulgent lines that some people may have trouble finding locally. For the housebound and full-time carers, it's definitely a site to bookmark.

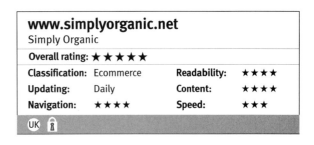

www.simplyorganic.net
Simply Organic

Overall rating: ★ ★ ★ ★			
Classification:	Ecommerce	**Readability:**	★ ★ ★ ★
Updating:	Daily	**Content:**	★ ★ ★ ★
Navigation:	★ ★ ★ ★	**Speed:**	★ ★ ★

Officially approved by the Soil Association, and based in New Covent Garden Market, Simply Organic delivers fresh organic produce and groceries direct to your door. With a range of over 1000 products, it is possible to do a very substantial shop from this site. The menu strip along the top of the homepage provides details of the company. To start shopping, head to the far right of the screen where the product categories are listed under Direct to the Aisles.

SPECIAL FEATURES

Homepage tells you straight away how soon your groceries can be delivered. At the checkout you can pick a different time if you like.

Fresh Fruit and Vegetables You can choose fruit and vegetables à la carte or order from a selection of convenient mixed boxes.

Fish The wild ocean fish, which are not allowed to be called organic, come from a supplier in Billingsgate market and are of a tremendously high quality.

Groceries For the healthy eater, Simply Organic's range includes both wholewheat and regular pastas, and breakfast cereals, including popular cereals from Jordans and Doves Farm, and Nature's Path organic millet flakes. A long-life milk section offers whole, semi-skimmed, and skimmed cows' milk varieties plus Provamel's excellent soya milks.

Chilled Foods   A choice of tofu brands is offered, plus vegetarian hot dogs, sausages, and frankfurters. Soya desserts are from Provamel and Soja Sun.

Infant contains a large selection of babyfood from the prestigious German brand Hipp, and British company Baby Organix. Also available are environmentally friendly nappies and Earth Friendly baby bodycare products.

Personal and Home Care features organic essential oils from Botanicus, Natracare feminine hygiene products, Green People and Nutique haircare, skincare and body wash products, plus Ecover washing up liquids, bleach and fabric conditioner.

News highlights the latest additions to the range, improvements to the site, interesting brands, and the occasional customer accolade.

Seasonal Offers is worth a look for special products or deals only available at certain times of the year.

OTHER FEATURES

Meat, wine and beer, organic gifts, gift certificates, company background information, and links to websites of manufacturers.

Simply Organic is a marvellous alternative to the major supermarkets, especially in terms of efficiency and order fulfilment.

www.snowandrock.com
Snow and Rock

Overall rating: ★ ★ ★ ★ ★			
Classification:	Ecommerce	Readability:	★ ★ ★ ★
Updating:	twice a year	Content:	★ ★ ★ ★
Navigation:	★ ★ ★ ★ ★	Speed:	★ ★ ★

UK 🔒

'Hi-energy' sports clothes and equipment are featured at this site for lovers of extreme activities and outdoor enthusiasts. The rest of us will get tired just looking at the pictures. You can choose whether you want to view the site in its regular or enhanced Flash version. After entering the site there is a brief explanation of how to shop there, but in order to make a purchase you have to take out free membership. The range is navigable from the menu panel at the left-hand side of the screen, and once within a section, bear in mind that there may be many more products in that category than at first appear – you may need to click on the View More arrows at the base of the screen.

SPECIAL FEATURES

X-Mountain Serious brands here include Gore, Lowe Alpine, and Patagonia, amongst others, and the wide range incorporates body warmers, jackets, shorts, biking jerseys, tops, and so on with all the key technological fabrics for wicking away all that sweat you're going to produce.

Active Lifestyle is the place to look for rugged clothes for hanging out but the brands are nonetheless the speciality names and not those found in every high street department store.

Summer Collection   Several of the cutting-edge surfwear manufacturers are featured here – Quicksilver, Billabong,

Rip Curl and No Fear. You'll find a load of sexy tops, shorts, and dresses for beach and about-town wear.

Protective Outerwear includes cuddly fleeces but also the hard-wearing jackets you need when positioned half way up a cold mountain. There is a wide range of price points covered.

Accessories encompasses high fashion sports watches and sunglasses plus tools, smalls, personal care, and first aid items for the genuinely outdoorsy.

Kids Here's what the best-dressed active children should be wearing, from groovy shirts and sandals for the beach to a full-body waterproof suit.

Footwear includes boots, sandals, socks, and a tremendous range of specialist rock shoes for feet planning a trip to rugged terrain, plus some casual fashion shoes. Also here are products for looking after both shoes and feet.

Climbing offers a wide range of specialist equipment including walking sticks, ice axes, harnesses, ropes, pulleys, and so on.

Travel & Trekking Not just sleeping bags, sweetie, but 'sleeping systems'. Also here, camping equipment, including food, cookers, water filters, lighting, insect repellent, a variety of tents, plus backpacks and bags.

OTHER FEATURES

Discussion forum, details of the Ace Races Challenge.

Active sports enthusiasts will already be familiar with this impressive range, but can now order products to be delivered to their door – a definite bonus if there is no branch locally.

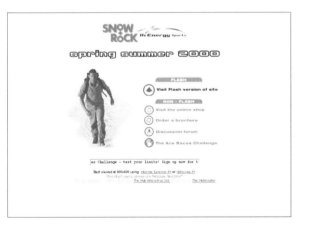

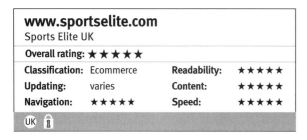

www.sportselite.com
Sports Elite UK

Overall rating: ★ ★ ★ ★ ★			
Classification:	Ecommerce	**Readability:**	★ ★ ★ ★ ★
Updating:	varies	**Content:**	★ ★ ★ ★ ★
Navigation:	★ ★ ★ ★ ★	**Speed:**	★ ★ ★ ★ ★

UK

You don't have to be an elite sports person or even an enthusiastic exerciser to appreciate this site. Click on the button on the entry page to take you through to the detailed homepage. You can search the site by keyword, size, price range, and colour, or navigate using the menu panel down the right of the screen that lists a wide variety of departments. Some particular products are highlighted at the centre of the page and you can click on the icon at the bottom of the page to view sale items.

SPECIAL FEATURES

Sale Items on our last visit included brilliant value half-price shoes and clothes. Colourways and sizes were limited, but not too much.

Ladies Sportswear is divided into brands including Reebok and Adidas, but items from other leading companies such as Nike and Ellesse are offered under the general heading of Top Brand. There is also a value section. We thought this brilliant, with an excellent selection of sizes, styles and colours we had not seen elsewhere. New, special offer, and seasonal items are highlighted.

Men's Sportswear offers a huge range of stylish shirts, jackets, sweat tops, tracksuits, bottoms and a wide range of brands including Fila, Umbro, Fred Perry, and loads more. Now what would be really cool is to offer the women this much choice...

Ladies Footwear Again, the range is impressive – it even includes comfy sports sandals – and the photography brilliant, but it would be useful here to have some advice on which shoes are good for which feet, particularly when it comes to the running shoes. At the moment it looks more like a collection of fashion shoes than sports shoes.

Weight Training includes a variety of home multi-gyms, some with steppers and cross-trainers to help you with at-home cardio workouts, plus weight sets and benches. The prices looked a little too reasonable...

Fitness Equipment features exercise cycles, treadmills and walkers, rowers and steppers, plus Slendertone machines and the excellent Tanita body fat monitoring scales.

OTHER FEATURES

Men's Footwear, Golf, Fishing, Football, and Cycling for men, women and children.

The photography is excellent, and the range of sizes and styles is better than most. This is a definite favourite, but more advice and information on products would be useful. Although the range is admirable, at times this company seems more like a fashion retailer than a sports retailer.

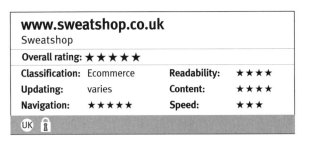

www.sweatshop.co.uk
Sweatshop

Overall rating: ★ ★ ★ ★ ★			
Classification:	Ecommerce	**Readability:**	★ ★ ★ ★
Updating:	varies	**Content:**	★ ★ ★ ★
Navigation:	★ ★ ★ ★ ★	**Speed:**	★ ★ ★

UK

Sweatshop claims to be the UK's biggest running, aerobics, and cross-training specialists, and as the homepage states, was voted retailer of the year for the last three years by readers of Athletics Weekly and Today's Runner. It was also voted best sports retailer by readers of Health and Fitness. The site takes a while to load, but is very easy to navigate using the row of pale blue buttons at the top of the screen.

SPECIAL FEATURES

Online Catalogue is divided into running, track and field, fitness, tennis, and sale sections. A variety of leading brands (Adidas, Nike, Saucony, New Balance) is offered, but certainly not all products from all companies. We liked the fact that the men's and women's running shoes section was divided into shoes for over-pronators, racing, off-road, and those people requiring extra support or cushioning. However, it was felt that Sweatshop missed a prime opportunity to offer a wide range of sizes in both shoes and clothing – the net is exactly where people requiring petite or large sizes want to turn, and a means by which companies can service them cost-effectively. We appreciated the sale section, too, although felt that many items offered were highly priced in the first place. There is a handy exercise-accessories section for buying items such as water bottles and heart rate monitors. We expect track and field sports people will find this very useful. You can also access a shop directory.

Advice Centre is a chat room for posting messages and asking questions – it's reasonably well attended but would be enhanced by some more professional input and advice to make it a better venue for fitness enthusiasts.

Sweatshop Information is a rather misleading title. This channel does include the company history and philosophy, but also offers a weekly training sheet to print out and details of some of the sophisticated fitness services offered by Sweatshop, such as the Nike lab lactate testing, a free sports injury clinic, and the Adidas foot scan which will help determine what running shoes you need to wear.

This is an excellent site but there is room for improvement, especially when it comes to catering for customers not in the typical size range – they need fitness clothing too and Sweatshop, if anyone, should be able to supply them.

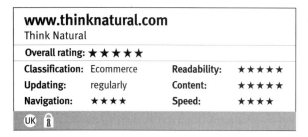

www.thinknatural.com
Think Natural

Overall rating: ★ ★ ★ ★ ★

Classification:	Ecommerce	Readability:	★ ★ ★ ★ ★
Updating:	regularly	Content:	★ ★ ★ ★ ★
Navigation:	★ ★ ★ ★	Speed:	★ ★ ★ ★

UK

Hertfordshire-based Think Natural was launched in the last quarter of 1999 by Emma Crowe and Carol Dukes, who aim both to educate people about natural health, and sell remedies. To this end the site features text from a Dorling Kindersley book on health, plus articles from journalists, natural health practitioners, and the high-profile columnist and author Dr Sarah Brewer.

The lively but somewhat bitty homepage offers many points of entry and means of searching. On the left are the two main menus that allow you to browse by type of therapy or by ailment (aches and pains, no smoking, and so on). Alternatively, search the site by keyword, take a look at the highlighted best sellers, or click on one of the subject-led articles.

SPECIAL FEATURES

Vitamins and Minerals Power Health, Health Aid, Vega, and FSC are among the top brands featured. Articles on dietary supplementation flash up to whet your appetite, for example 'Get zinc-wise', 'Get healthy with royal jelly', 'Why you need vitamin B6', 'Bone up with calcium' and 'Check your folic acid levels'.

Herbs and Medicinal A search here for a bunion remedy turned up an article by the esteemed Dr Sarah Brewer, who recommended vitamin C, evening primrose oil, aloe vera gel, and a hot epsom salt foot bath. Agnus castus was recommended to help 'regain your balance'. You could also 'take the itch out of psoriasis', read up on 'natural aphrodisiacs' or find out how to 'spring clean your system'.

Aromatherapy includes kits for conditions and situations such as the Essential Birth kit, first aid oils, skin soothers, and oils to help digestion. Leading brands featured include Tisserand, HealthAid, and Absolute Aromas, and there are some difficult-to-find varieties such as the premium-priced jasmine oil, plus popular essences like basil, lavender, and ylang-ylang.

Natural Bodycare Click on the articles for advice on moisturising and the site's plan to 'banish cellulite forever'. Tempting products for sale include willowherb, bluebell, and yarrow foam bath, citrus toothpaste, and Soothe Aromabubble from stylish Nelson and Russell.

Homeopathic Remedies Amongst the well-known brands available here are Nelson's, Weleda, New Era Biochemic and Ainsworths. There are some good articles, too.

Flower Remedies come from Ainsworths. If you don't know the particular remedy you need, click on one of the feelings you may be experiencing. Suggestions include 'dead to life', 'lonely heart', 'rise from rock bottom', 'if only I could be certain', 'don't feel the fear', and 'sensitive flower'.

Gifts change, and may include a luxury bath set for lovers with bath fizz and scented candle, or a series of herbal preparations for problem skin from Annemarie Borlind, a company manufacturing skincare products 'for the natural generation'.

Specials There are usually many special offers such as two for the price of one. Prices include postage and packing.

OTHER FEATURES

Information about the company, contact details, contributor biographies, jobs, and suppliers.

A very good shopping and information site with lots of pithy, easy-to-digest articles on a wide variety of subjects.

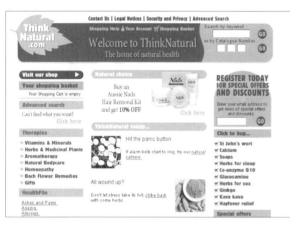

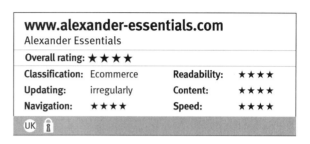

www.alexander-essentials.com
Alexander Essentials

Overall rating: ★ ★ ★ ★			
Classification:	Ecommerce	**Readability:**	★ ★ ★ ★
Updating:	irregularly	**Content:**	★ ★ ★ ★
Navigation:	★ ★ ★ ★	**Speed:**	★ ★ ★ ★

UK

This specialist aromatherapy site has a vast list of essential oils and related products at sensible prices. Alexander Essentials is a member of the Guild of Master Craftsmen and pride themselves on 'offering only the best'. The company often buys from small specialist international suppliers. The site is excellent for hard-to-find oils and related products not stocked at high street chemists or health food shops, but you do need to know what you are looking for and why. Unusually, the company offers many different sized bottles so is particularly good for trial sizes and bulk users, and it boasts many practitioners amongst its clients. The prices exclude VAT, but postage and packing is free to UK addresses. To enter, simply click on one of the categories listed on the homepage.

SPECIAL FEATURES

Special Offers features discounts on a wide variety of selected oils and special discounts on orders of two bottles or more. On a recent visit, Bulgarian rose absolute (widely thought to be the finest), was being offered at £15 for 5ml; and 30ml of lavender essential oil was £10. A litre of sweet almond carrier oil was £9.50, and reduced to £8.50 each for two or more bottles.

Essential Oils and Aromatherapy Products is a more comprehensive section than the name suggests. Along with alphabetically listed essential and carrier oils, there are also products for sale, including books, potpourri, floral waters, and soaps. There's also an online guide to basic essential oil use that includes information on country of origin, an explanation of market forces issues, and advice on finding an aromatherapist.

Herbal Body Care lists items such as lip balms, hair conditioners, treatment shampoos, handcare, fragrance-free products, mens' and baby ranges, facial cleansers, toners, and lotions. Natural soaps include some charming combinations such as bergamot and orange, grapefruit and juniper, neroli and lemongrass, or teatree with eucalyptus. Simply fragrant rather than therapeutic are the banana and vanilla, rose and cinnamon, coconut ice, or mango and apricot soaps. Scroll down further to the complexion treatment soaps such as carrot with wheatgerm for dry skins, or orchid oil and cocoa butter soap for normal skins.

Total Clean is a particular face and body cleanser the company is highlighting. It seems extraordinarily versatile.

What this site lacks in trendy design is admirably compensated for by range, expertise, and ease of navigation, and it is a joy to shop from.

www.allcures.com
All Cures

Overall rating: ★ ★ ★ ★			
Classification:	Ecommerce	Readability:	★ ★ ★ ★
Updating:	Daily	Content:	★ ★ ★ ★ ★
Navigation:	★ ★ ★ ★	Speed:	★ ★ ★ ★ ★

UK 🔒

Despite its dotcom URL, this is a British company and claims to be 'the first fully operational online pharmacy in the UK'. The simple splash page is divided into the main departments listed below. You simply pick the one you want to enter first and can access the other sections once inside the site using the navigational strip across the top of the page or the menu panel down the left-hand side of the screen.

SPECIAL FEATURES

All Beauty Products aims to have everything men and women need to keep them looking and smelling good. When you have chosen this section a range of featured products will appear on the main part of the screen. To browse the aisles in a sensible fashion you need to scroll down to the bottom of the page and choose by product category. The women's fragrance section was not particularly exciting in terms of range, although several perfumes were being sold at a discount of £5 or more.

All Pharmacy offers a prescription dispensing service for NHS and private prescriptions. Scroll down to the bottom of the page to browse the aisles by product category; alternatively you can select brands from the pulldown menu to the right.

All Toiletries We thought this range practical but unexciting.

There is a comprehensive selection of treatment shampoos for those with irritated scalps.

All Ternative covers a range of homeopathy, aromatherapy, vitamin supplements, flower remedies, plus anti-smoking and slimming aids. You can browse sections such as Herbal Remedies by condition (menopaude, stress, catarrh etc) as well as brand.

All Health-info is a source of health and medical information with text supplied by NetDoctor.co.uk (see p. ??). The News section, which is accessed from the menu panel at the left of the screen, is a series of links to articles on major news sites around the world, including the BBC, CNN, Bangkok Post and Hindustan Times(!). The Health Features are lengthy, informative, and have appropriate contact details of support and information groups at the bottom of each page.

FAQs There is an extremely long list of frequently asked questions, covering health (and photographic) issues as well as online shopping, presented in a pulldown menu. It is a good ready-reckoner of problems with concise, to-the-point answers.

Ask the Expert requires site registration but allows you to consult with the pharmacists at All Cures in private via email.

Links There was an extensive list of information resources categorised by ailment and situation however none of the links we clicked on worked and key sites were missing from the subject categories.

OTHER FEATURES
Photographic development, gifts, special offers.

A good online pharmacy for regular items but, like Pharmacy 2U, it lacks the exciting or unusual items that could distinguish it from your local high-street chemist.

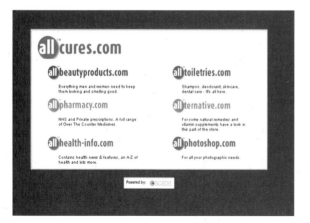

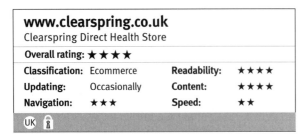

www.clearspring.co.uk
Clearspring Direct Health Store

Overall rating: ★ ★ ★ ★

Classification:	Ecommerce	**Readability:**	★ ★ ★ ★
Updating:	Occasionally	**Content:**	★ ★ ★ ★
Navigation:	★ ★ ★	**Speed:**	★ ★

UK 🔒

Clearspring is a long-established importer-retailer of Japanese and macrobiotic foods, as well as other health products. Although they have products to push, health claims tend to be backed up by research findings. On first arrival at the site, the shopping program can take a while to load. Enter via the icon on the opening page, and choose from the menu, a series of pebbles around the top right of the screen. The pages are very long and, once at the end, you usually have to scroll back up to the top to change sections.

SPECIAL FEATURES

Books offers a small selection of speciality titles not readily found elsewhere, including books on sprouting, cooking with vegetarian proteins, and sea vegetables. More general themes are covered too in the Self-Healing Cookbook, Culinary Treasures of Japan, and Vegetarian Classics.

Bodycare is the place for Clearspring's organic toothpaste, scented ear candles, natural cleansers, tonics and creams, aloe vera shampoo, shower gel, and so on.

Kitchenware includes the macrobiotic cook's essential pressure cooker, plus Japanese equipment such as knives, sushi mats, suribachi, ginger graters, a pickle press, and a sprouting jar for all those healthy beansprouts you'll be eating.

Macrobiotic Specialities lists sushi pickles including ginger, daikon, garlic with ume, and cucumber, and there are ingredients like kuzu (starch for thickening), umeboshi plums and purée, ume shiso sprinkle, wasabi, dried lotus root and daikon, and a fascinating dried tofu from Japan.

Miso links to an article explaining what miso is, how to use it, and its medicinal benefits. Several of the eight varieties offered for sale are organic, and the company has a choice of instant miso soups.

Pasta includes regular and gluten free pastas such as buckwheat spirals, corn and spinach rigati, rice and millet spirals, and rice and soya shells.

Seasonings Here you will find fine Japanese ingredients such as red plum seasoning, brown rice vinegar, toasted sesame oil and mirin, which can all be used as alternatives to salt.

Sea Vegetables This is a superior and extremely comprehensive range from Europe, the USA, and Japan, including a mixed 'sea salad' of dulse, sea lettuce, and nori from Breton. There is a link to explanatory articles on sea vegetables and the varieties available.

Soya and Vegetable Products includes hard-to-find tempeh, plus organic vegetarian ready meal products including tofu ravioli, seitan bolognese, and ratatouille.

Sweets are unnervingly healthy here. Choose from carob chews, sour plum sweets, brown rice sweet crunch, various types of brown rice crackers flavoured with things like tamari and sesame, plus English water crackers, malt digestives, and carob biscuits.

Recipes include several taken from books by esteemed macrobiotic cook Montse Bradford. Obviously the aim is to get you using the products, so there are dishes made from miso, noodles, and seaweed, plus many for one of the company's high-profile brands, Rice Dream, an alternative to cow's milk. At the bottom of each recipe the ingredients needed can be automatically added to your shopping basket. There is a good section within the noodle recipes, to help you tell your soba from your yagitori soba.

Press Releases There is some interesting information here, such as details of Japanese research into the health benefits of miso. It's thought the high consumption of it has helped protect people there from radiation poisoning.

List of Suppliers aims to let you know if Clearspring products are available from health food shops in your area, but many of them are without addresses and phone numbers.

OTHER FEATURES

Very many other products are listed in categories such as tea and drinks, malted syrups, desserts, nut butter, organic oils, and pulses. There's also news, company details, a section for wholesale enquiries, and links to other health food businesses, macrobiotic organisations, and the Macrobiotic Ring, which Clearspring owns.

A great site to know if your local area suffers from the lack of a good healthfood store, or if you have a particular interest in the macrobiotic lifestyle.

www.sweatybetty.com
Sweaty Betty

Overall rating: ★ ★ ★ ★

Classification:	Ecommerce	Readability:	★ ★ ★ ★
Updating:	Occasionally	Content:	★ ★ ★ ★
Navigation:	★ ★ ★	Speed:	★ ★

UK

Sweaty Betty is a small chain of sportswear stores established in 1998 with the aim of making stylish activewear for women more readily available. This is a very friendly, sexy site with moving images and funky drawings but no immediately visible words to help you navigate. It takes quite a while to load but is generally worth the wait. Once the images of the five girls appear, hold your cursor over each one and wait for the names of the various sections to come up. Choose a department, then use the cute arrows to scroll up and down the range. Click on any items you wish to view. When they have loaded, click on the picture of the eyeball to view in more detail and to read the sizing and colour information.

SPECIAL FEATURES

Anywear The most exciting section, with several tempting mix-and-match outfits, generally premium priced. Pilates gear features because it is stylish enough to be worn away from the reformer or mat work class. There is also an innovative alternative to leggings and a big baggy T-shirt for those of us wanting to keep our hips covered.

Beachwear Lots of bikinis, a few one-pieces, plus pareos and nice sundresses.

Snowwear Only a fleecy jacket was on offer on our visit – the season was over.

Sweatwear Several good items are featured; however, the site makes the common mistake of thinking that everyone who exercises wants to wear teeny outfits to show off their hot bod. There were no short-sleeved shirts, for example, amongst the many vests and bra-style tops, and the only option for modest women had strappy shoulders that would make flabby arms look larger than life.

Accessories A disappointing section that included only flip-flops – they promise to expand this range with bags, and so on, in future.

OTHER FEATURES

What the Papers Say, The Place (their outlets) and The Story (the mission statement and company history).

A very exciting site with great attitude but it would serve women even better by catering more carefully to females of all sizes and not just the fit, sexy ones. They plan to expand the site to include health and fitness information, something we look forward to.

www.clickchs.co.uk
Christopher's Home Shopping

Overall rating: ★ ★ ★

Classification:	Ecommerce	Readability:	★ ★ ★
Updating:	Varies	Content:	★ ★ ★
Navigation:	★ ★ ★ ★	Speed:	★ ★ ★

UK 🔒

It's difficult not to be attracted by this beautifully illustrated site. The owners certainly seem to have their hearts in the right place, as they are keen to support artisan producers and organic, natural products. Not everything here is organic (though it is GM free), nor is everything healthy in the traditional sense – it's a site that is likely to appeal to gourmets, too. It is based on a theme of several small village shops and, for all its technological advancement, on good old-fashioned home delivery. To begin shopping, try really hard not to let your mouse click on the range of truffles from The Chocolate Society (which are the best you can buy) and instead move to the organic fruit and vegetable boxes, natural health remedies, or something else really virtuous.

SPECIAL FEATURES

Natural Health Remedies includes the usual flower remedies and essential oils. More interesting, however, is the Kombucha range of drinks, skin creams, and animal products. Kombucha is considered to be one of the great elixirs of life, said to relieve symptoms of eczema and asthma, help sufferers of ME and arthritis, improve liver function, cleanse blood, detoxify – all those things your GP will probably pooh-pooh but which Harold Tietze, a medical herbalist, has been attempting to prove.

Organic Fruit and Veg is based on box delivery with several sizes available of fruit and veg boxes including an extra-large fruit box for £16 and a large veg box for £12. We would prefer some more insight into what the boxes may contain; however, some guidance is given on sizing: the large veg box will apparently feed a family of six for a week.

The Essential Larder contains 100 per cent organic foods and groceries such as bodycare, pet and household products. More detailed product information, pictures and details of the brands supplying the website would be welcome here.

Butcher   Meat lovers will thrill to this selection, which includes free range poultry, game, exotic meats, English Longhorn beef, rare-breed pork, Yorkshire lamb, and venison.

OTHER FEATURES

Wines, seafood, gourmet ready meals, bread, coffee, dairy produce, smoked produce, and much more.

The site was newly launched on our visit, and early teething troubles are likely to be ironed out quickly. Many products here are not widely available from other internet or mail order retailers, so this site is certainly worth visiting.

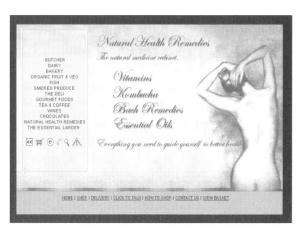

www.healthfoodstore.co.uk
Health Food Store

Overall rating: ★ ★ ★			
Classification:	Ecommerce	**Readability:**	★ ★ ★
Updating:	Infrequently	**Content:**	★ ★ ★
Navigation:	★ ★ ★ ★	**Speed:**	★ ★ ★ ★

UK 🔒

The company behind this attractive site is based in Gloucestershire, and promises free postage and packaging for orders over £30, which, let's face it, with the cost of vitamins and minerals these days is a pretty easy target to reach. Click on the daisy to enter the store, which promises 'all your online health food needs'. You can search the site by keyword, choosing one of the daisies from the menu strip across the top of the page, or read information sheets by selecting one of the subjects listed in the panel down the left side of the screen. To begin shopping, click on the shop-front icons at the centre of the homepage.

SPECIAL FEATURES

Information contains the site's links, plus a basic guide to vitamins and minerals, herbal products, and aromatherapy oils. It's brief, to-the-point reference material rather than an enjoyable read, but nevertheless a useful touchstone when shopping.

Food Supplements, Vitamins and Minerals contains several leading brands including Solgar, Quest, and Blackmores.

Giftstore includes a range of knick-knacks, candles, natural soaps and perfumes, aromatherapy vaporisers, incense, and so on.

Essential Oils and Fragrances breaks down oils into warming, relaxing, stimulating, and refreshing varieties and includes a list of oils to avoid during pregnancy plus other warnings regarding safe usage. Song of India is a favoured brand and there are several unusual varieties such as thujka wood, tagette and sugandh-mantri. The Natural by Nature brand is also available.

Sport and Fitness features the Weider and Nutrisport ranges of sports dietary supplements, which are of particular interest to weight lifters and body builders.

Herbal Remedies come from the respected companies Potters (elixirs and natural cold remedies), and Bach, the leading flower remedy brand.

Personal Care Products include items from Nelsons, Tom's of Maine, Dead Sea Magik, and tea tree oils from Thursday Plantation.

Vegetarians is not a shopping section, but contains listings of ingredients that may be found in food, supplements, or personal products that are derived from animals and which vegetarians may want to avoid.

Hayfever contains information about this common allergy, which it is claimed affects 15 to 20 percent of the British population. Unfortunately the section seems to focus more on what it is, rather than effective means of avoiding it.

E numbers is a basic guide to, you guessed it, E numbers.

OTHER FEATURES

Forum, book store, special offers, pet care, household, conversion chart, and a well-considered selection of links to medical, government, media, and health product manufacturers.

The name is a bit misleading – it's a health shop rather than a health food store, but this site is very easy to use.

www.humankinetics.com
Human Kinetics

Overall rating: ★ ★ ★			
Classification:	Ecommerce	Readability:	★ ★ ★ ★
Updating:	Irregular	Content:	★ ★ ★ ★
Navigation:	★ ★ ★ ★	Speed:	★ ★ ★

US 🔒

Human Kinetics is an outstanding publisher of health and fitness books, journals, videos, software, distance education, and so on, aimed primarily at the fitness professional and serious enthusiast. As they put it: 'In today's world, survival of the fittest means survival of the best informed.'

On the homepage, click on books under Product Center in the left-hand menu panel, or if you want to look around a little, select one of the other channels highlighted on the main section of the page. The pull-down menu under Select a Subject is not for searching the site, but leads you to the various sections of the company's academic/professional channel. Human Kinetics has a British distributor who will post the items to you, and you can click on UK underneath your chosen product to convert prices to British pounds.

SPECIAL FEATURES

Books More than 100 books a year are printed by the company. Some are textbooks, and very scholarly, but many are suitable for keen exercisers and amateur sports enthusiasts. This section offers a search facility to help you navigate the huge range. Browse by subject from the pull-down menu or search for a book by keyword, title, ISBN number, or author. Click on Browse by Subject and you will be presented with two long lists, one for the academic or professional, the other for the consumer. Subjects run from Aerobics to Wrestling and Yoga, via every sport you can think of including cheerleading. There are two books and a video just on jumping rope. Human Kinetics offers several good books on exercise psychology and motivation to help you muster the go get 'em mindset of top professional athletes, also very good books on exercising specific parts of the body. Look down beneath the blurb and author information and you'll find a complete list of contents and media reviews, which is very helpful when making a decision whether to buy.

Videos are, unfortunately, available only in the American PAL format.

OTHER FEATURES

Links are given to various sports associations and academic bodies, and other sections include journals, software, distance education, academic gateways, and faculty center.

If you're into a sport like lacrosse or snowshoeing, you probably know about this excellent company already, because few others cover speciality fitness areas in such depth. Yet there are many good books here for people who simply want to take up cycling, improve their golf game, or tone up their abs.

www.proactive-health.co.uk
Proactive Health

Overall rating: ★ ★ ★			
Classification:	Ecommerce	Readability:	★ ★ ★ ★
Updating:	Irregular	Content:	★ ★ ★
Navigation:	★ ★ ★ ★	Speed:	★ ★ ★ ★

UK

Proactive Health was formed in 1992 to supply trade and consumers with fitness equipment. They are serious about exercise and rightfully remind us that 'buying from Proactive Health Limited is not a workout!', although it is about buying major 'investment pieces' of exercise equipment. From the homepage, click on the Site Contents pull-down menu at the lower right of the page.

SPECIAL FEATURES

Online Store of more than 700 items featuring a section dedicated to Reebok goods. To search the main Proactive section, select a category of equipment from the pull-down menu in the centre of the page. There are 34 sections including instructors' products, and large pieces of equipment such as rowing machines, as well as general consumer lines like exercise tubes. Delivery charges are a little high, although next day delivery is possible if orders are placed before noon. The company would do well to take a tip from other mail-order suppliers and put a ceiling on delivery charges, or failing that, offer free delivery on orders over a specified amount. As it is, the more items you order, the more the price goes up.

Help is where you'll find the answers to frequently asked questions on shipping, delivery, security, and so on.

Powerblock links through to a separate site for a particular weight lifting product designed for serious enthusiasts.

OTHER FEATURES

Virtual Club, Promotions and News sections were under construction as we went to press. Links are given to Reebok, York, Polar, Life Fitness, and other manufacturers of fitness equipment, plus some gyms.

Proactive Health offers an excellent range and are a very good option for those people shopping for fitness equipment who cannot get to a sports store. For city-dwellers, however, the excessive delivery charges may make this site an uneconomical choice, especially as the equipment is not offered at a discount in the manner of many other online retailers.

OTHER SITES OF INTEREST

Click Mango
www.clickmango.com
Don't forget that Click Mango (see p. 67 for full review) offers a brilliant range of rare health and beauty products by mail order. Top brands include Liz Earle skincare, and Bharti Vytas products

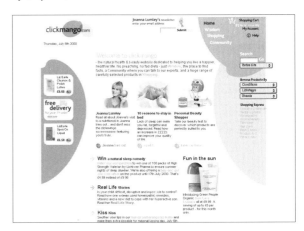

eNutrition
www.eNutrition.com
Given the impressive standard of UK sites such as Think Natural and Nutravida, it's not really necessary to purchase health products online from America. However, this is a good site, featuring interesting articles for sports and fitness enthusiasts including interviews with noted superbodies about their dietary and lifestyle habits.

Vitamin Shoppe

www.vitaminshoppe.com

This American company sponsors the site of complementary/integrative health practitioner Dr Andrew Weil (see p. 48) and offers a range of quality products.

Lakeland Limited

www.lakelandlimited.co.uk

A handy address for mail-order kitchenware. There are some terrific products for the healthy cook, including an olive oil spray pump, which gives pans a fine film of oil without the yukky smell of propellants. Also available are several different types of steamer, non-stick pans, bakeware and utensils, a glass fat separator for low-fat gravies, nonstick baking parchment, and many styles of fun boxes for taking healthy packed lunches to work.

Cucina Direct

www.cucinadirect.co.uk

Cucina Direct has around seven years experience in selling kitchenware by mail order. They sell state-of-the-art nonstick

cookware from German company SKK, and the impressive Le Pentole sets of steaming pots. The equipment is pricey, but highly recommended for many years of satisfying healthy cooking. SKK pans are also available from www.divertimenti.com.

Waitrose

www.waitrose.com

Unlike the sites of other large supermarket retailers, Waitrose is very easy to access and order from. The organic fruit and vegetable boxes come highly recommended: excellent quality and convenient packaging, plus prompt delivery, though it may require a half-day-at-home commitment.

Chapter 7

men's health

Men are renowned for being hypochondriacs but at the same time often exhibit a tremendous reluctance when it comes to visiting a doctor to try and sort things out. It can also be the case that the very things that make someone a man – that is, the genitalia – are the most embarrassing and frightening things to have to discuss when there is a problem.

This no doubt is a contributing factor in the lack of awareness about serious diseases like testicular cancer, which is the most common form of cancer in young men. Rates are doubling every 20 years, but it has a disturbingly low awareness rating amongst 15–34-year-old males.

Another reason to ensure that men find it easier to access, understand and deal with their health issues quickly is that long-term problems with the sex organs can lead to other serious conditions such as depression.

Thank goodness for the internet. It allows you to read about and discuss private health matters as it needs to be done – in private – and yet you can also share experiences of ailments and treatments with other sufferers. In addition to the useful URLs in this chapter, you will find many good men's health channels within the sites featured in the general medical section, and excellent information at www.embarrassingproblems.co.uk.

www.boots-men.co.uk
Boots Men

Overall rating: ★ ★ ★ ★			
Classification:	Information	**Readability:**	★ ★ ★ ★
Updating:	Varies	**Content:**	★ ★ ★ ★
Navigation:	★ ★ ★ ★ ★	**Speed:**	★ ★ ★ ★ ★

UK 🛈

'This is the essential guide to men's grooming and health' proclaims this site from the high street health and beauty retailer Boots. On arrival you find that two features are promoted in the centre of the screen and these change each time you re-load the page. Navigation is simple, through the collection of links to site sections, or 'zones', in the top right of the screen. You can also register so that the site navigation is re-organised and your favourite areas brought to the top. The zones are enhanced through Flash-based animations.

SPECIAL FEATURES

Health and Fitness offers an interactive guide to vitamins and minerals and articles dealing with a broad range of subjects including life after nicotine, hangover cures and ins, general fitness and how to get a good night's sleep. Features here, as elsewhere, are short and to the point, providing only the most significant facts.

Fragrance Here we found an animation that described five ways of keeping you smelling fragrant. On clicking the mannequin's boxer shorts we were told 'Fresh pants: Need we say more? Change your underwear at least once a day'. This no-nonsense approach is carried through with three articles concerning beating body odour, dealing with smelly feet and the best fragrances to use for a date. Specific products are rarely mentioned and there is no direct opportunity to buy. If its ecommerce you're looking for, a visit to the main Boots site http://www.boots.co.uk/ is necessary – but you can simply click on the link.

Grooming Just two articles here during our last visit. Both 'A Man for the Big Occasion' and 'Groom to Manoeuvre' recommended that men pluck their eyebrows, especially if they meet in the middle. Ouch.

Hair and Body offers tips on removing unwanted body hair, dying hair, and top eye care tips. Another feature, 'Coming clean', attempts to settle the argument over which is better – bath or shower? In the end they call it a draw.

Shaving Here we found an illustrated guide to the perfect wet shave and a comparison of wet and dry shaving. Given the small amount of material in this and the above two categories, we felt the three zones could be merged into one. But perhaps there is more to come.

Skincare argues there's more to a good facial regime than just soap and water. You will also find information on moisturising for men, details of how to be safe in the sun, and ways of dealing with spots and blackheads.

Links to the online store, plus occasional links to other sites as a source of further information at the end of articles.

OTHER FEATURES

What's New, information about the Boots Men stores and current in-store promotions.

This is what you expect from one of the UK's leading health and beauty retailers – a slick and professional site full of useful tips that a lot of men will find handy.

www.gmhp.demon.co.uk
Gay Men's Health Wiltshire and Swindon

Overall rating: ★ ★ ★ ★			
Classification:	IHomepage	**Readability:**	★ ★ ★ ★ ★
Updating:	Frequently	**Content:**	★ ★ ★ ★
Navigation:	★ ★ ★ ★	**Speed:**	★ ★ ★ ★

UK

This site may be the work of a gay men's health project in Wiltshire, but its usefulness extends much further. The fact this site is a comprehensive resource of significant relevance to gay men and health workers is evident the moment you arrive on its homepage, which consists mainly of text links to content. The language used once you go below the homepage is often explicit. 'With the threat of HIV and AIDS,' the site warns visitors, 'it is necessary to use very blunt language and imagery that can be easily understood by all those who need to read it.' To navigate the site, click on the links on the pale blue menu panel down the left hand side of the screen, or read through the contents of the homepage and click on the highlighted features that interest you.

SPECIAL FEATURES

About Gay Men's Health This section details the history of the project and introduces visitors to the project's workers. You can also find out why the site uses strong language and sexual imagery.

What We Offer explains the services the project provides in the Wiltshire area. Provided you live in the area you can also order online free condoms and information packs here. 'Straight' Talk features articles from the project's newsletter, which you may download completely as Acrobat files if desired, or click on the headlines of the featured article to read online. Topics covered range from the political to the personal and practical, for example 'Section 28: the Reality and Truth of the Law', 'The Homosexual Age of Consent', 'Helping Gay Pupils', 'Exploring Gay Relationships', 'A Word from the Citizen's Advice Bureau' and 'Helping Self-Esteem'

Online Guides This is where you will find most of the explicit material. In-depth advice is given covering a selection of health matters including safe sex, coming out and staying out, STDs, and hepatitis. We also found two guides for GPs and general practice staff that both cover working with gay and bisexual men. Some guides are available in Adobe Acrobat format for printing.

The Directory offers information about gay men's projects and support organisations in Wiltshire and throughout the UK. There is also the web guide, which gives links to sites covering Gay and bisexual life, and HIV and AIDs.

Other Groups is an introduction to the other local organisations that the project supports.

OTHER FEATURES

Site newsletter.

This impressive site is comprehensive and well produced. Gay men and the health practitioners who work with them will find much to offer.

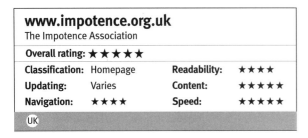

www.impotence.org.uk
The Impotence Association

Overall rating: ★ ★ ★ ★ ★			
Classification:	Homepage	Readability:	★ ★ ★ ★
Updating:	Varies	Content:	★ ★ ★ ★ ★
Navigation:	★ ★ ★ ★	Speed:	★ ★ ★ ★ ★

UK

The Impotence Association (also known as the ImpoAssociation) is a registered charity and was formed in 1995 to help sufferers and raise awareness of the condition. The site is modern, attractive and relatively easy to navigate, with some exceptions. It was built thanks to a grant from Pfizer, the makers of Viagra, but this does not affect the quality of information available within. To begin your research, click on one of the categories listed down the centre of the green and purple screen. While visiting the site, be sure to read the flashing comments from sufferers that appear on the screen from time to time – from the corner of the eye they may seem like a design affectation, but in fact are interesting and comforting.

SPECIAL FEATURES

Patient Information Leaflets offers six well-written and informative articles that may be read online. Topics include 'Impotence explained', 'Would a woman recognise the signs?', and 'Sexual difficulties in gay men'. Each article is broken into a number of questions such as 'What causes erectile dysfunction?'. Unfortunately, the only way to read an entire article is to click on a question, read the answer, go back to the article's main index, click on another question, and so on. You cannot read from start to finish in one go.

Questions and Answers This area introduces the Impotence Association and its history. It also provides some basic information about impotence such as the causes and methods of treatment, but the Patient Information Leaflets offer more detail.

Online Survey Here men suffering from impotence, or their partners, are invited to provide some details of their condition. The association hopes that the results from this anonymous questionnaire will enable them to 'know more about the number of men suffering from impotence, the treatments initiated, and how the condition affects people's lives.'

News Update provides the latest news about the Impotence Association and its activities, with hot topics such as 'Since the Launch of Viagra' highlighted with a flashing 'new' icon. It's an informative section: did you know that the British Medical Association estimates 120,000 men in their 30s and 40s suffer impotence as a direct result of smoking? You can also read a select number of features from their newsletter 'One in Ten' and browse letters from impotence sufferers. In response to enquiries from helpline callers, they have posted a list of complementary therapy associations who sufferers can contact for details of local practitioners who may be able to offer help with individual cases.

Supporting the IA invites visitors to make a donation or become a friend of the Association.

OTHER FEATURES

Details of the Impotence Helpline number and its service.

Whilst this site is let down in part by poor navigation, you will nonetheless find a great deal of information about impotence and currently available treatments.

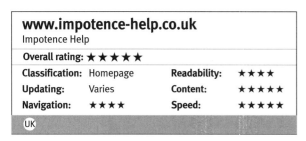

www.impotence-help.co.uk
Impotence Help

Overall rating: ★ ★ ★ ★ ★			
Classification:	Homepage	**Readability:**	★ ★ ★
Updating:	Varies	**Content:**	★ ★ ★ ★ ★
Navigation:	★ ★ ★ ★	**Speed:**	★ ★ ★ ★ ★

UK

You could be forgiven for raising an eyebrow the moment you discover this site is sponsored by Schwarz Pharma, a pharmaceutical company that produces a number of drugs for the treatment and diagnosis of erectile dysfunction (impotence or ED). In fact, the site honestly concentrates on informing visitors about the condition, which is said to affect 20 per cent of the UK male population between the ages of 40–65. The site is based on frames with the navigation being found on the left-hand side of the screen.

SPECIAL FEATURES

What is Impotence Illustrations and graphs accompany this explanation of impotence, its causes and risk factors and treatments. As the unattributed quotes from sufferers reveal: 'I thought I was alone – but now I realise this is a very common problem.'

Patient Stories Four sufferers explain their experience of having the condition and there follows a comment from a doctor, continuing the discussion about various forms of treatment. Site visitors are invited to share their stories too, in the hope that they may help others – you can do this by clicking on the relevant button here.

Your Visit to the Doctor This excellent section explains what to expect when you first consult your GP about erectile dysfunction. There is a list of typical questions you will be asked, an outline of the elements of the physical examination and other tests they may wish you to take, brief details of the treatments they may prescribe, and hints as to the lifestyle changes they may ask you to make – such as giving up smoking and cutting down on alcohol. Impotence can have emotional or psychological causes, so there is also information here on psychosexual counselling, too.

Frequently Asked Questions include 'Where should I go for the best treatment?', 'If I have to have surgery, will I have to pay for this?', 'What if my treatment doesn't work?', and 'Is there any such thing as the male menopause?'. The range of issues covered is impressive, but we felt the answers to the questions were just a little too brief, although they are clearly written and informative.

TV Doctor Mark Porter's Help Page This offers little but an explanation that the aim of the website is to help you 'set out on the path to seek the medical advice and treatment that you need'. There is the opportunity to download a five-page document written by Mark Porter and provided in Adobe Acrobat format, but this merely summarises the information provided elsewhere on the site.

Links Include The British Diabetic Association, The Men's Health section of healthcentre.org.uk and the Prostate Help Association at www.personal.u-net.com

OTHER FEATURES

Guest Book.

If you can find your way through the rather confusing frame-based navigation, you will find this site an informative guide to impotence.

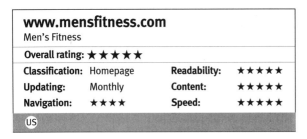

www.mensfitness.com

Men's Fitness

Overall rating: ★ ★ ★ ★ ★			
Classification:	Homepage	**Readability:**	★ ★ ★ ★ ★
Updating:	Monthly	**Content:**	★ ★ ★ ★ ★
Navigation:	★ ★ ★ ★	**Speed:**	★ ★ ★ ★ ★
US			

This American offering is part of the Fitness Online network of sites and provides around six articles a month from the current issue of Men's Fitness magazine. The latest features to be added are highlighted in the middle of the homepage, and during our last visit the selection was headed by 'Less Press, Bigger Chest', which explains 'How to improve your bench overnight without – well, almost without – bench-pressing'. This was supported by a heavily-illustrated step-by-step six-week workout. Usually the site does the decent thing and warns visitors that the image-laden workout may take a substantial time to download.

SPECIAL FEATURES

Training You will find workout and weight training features such as 'Less Press, Bigger Chest' in here. This section, like the others mentioned below, brings together previously-published articles on topics such as losing your love handles and building a better back. You won't find everything the magazine has published, but the guys here are some of the best and most authoritative in the field (or gym).

Nutrition One of the most fascinating articles here concerned 'The Dirty Dozen' – 12 fatty foods. The leading dish was KFC Extra Crispy Breast and Wing, which apparently contains 690 calories and 43 grams of fat. According to the article, the way to burn this off is to 'run

five-and-a-half miles at an eight-minute-per-mile pace.' Or to 'climb a steep rock face for 47 minutes.' Another article informed us that a survey carried out last year found the fattest city in America to be Philadelphia – home of cream cheese. The fittest city was San Diego.

Health Browse this section for features on diverse topics such as the power of the mind, the symptoms of concussion, and how to get rid of acne.

Sex & Behavior You know what to expect: '5 body parts that make women drool', 'Hold your fire', and 'Hard thinking'. Need we go on?

Sports & Adventure covers how to get fit through sports such as mountain biking, urban kayaking and orienteering. There's also advice on protective clothing for indoor racquet sports and the opportunity to 'learn what some of the world's top athletes do to sharpen their focus in the gym'.

Gear pulls together selected product reviews from previous issues of Men's Fitness. There is no direct opportunity to buy the items featured, which include headwear, eyewear, baggage, trainers and running shoes.

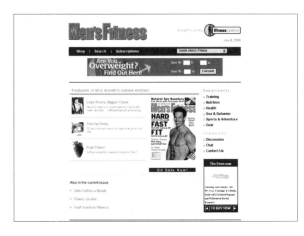

Links To Fitnessonline.com, which provides the site, and to the supplier of the Men's Fitness marketplace shopping section.

OTHER FEATURES

Discussion, chat.

A pleasant and attractive site, which is worthy of a monthly visit, if only to chuckle once again at the list of America's fattest cities.

www.the-penis.com
The Penis

Overall rating: ★ ★ ★ ★			
Classification:	Enthusiast	Readability:	★ ★ ★
Updating:	Irregular	Content:	★ ★ ★ ★
Navigation:	★ ★ ★ ★	Speed:	★ ★ ★ ★

US

It's difficult not to smirk that the Penis.com is produced by an enthusiast: however, in practice this is a useful information and gateway site for those with problems in that area, or uncertainties about what is normal. The range of information it deals with is comprehensive and more than compensates for the lack of fine design.

The homepage offers a menu strip across the top, with a general introduction to the site below. Scroll right down to see the recommended sites of the month and a version of a site map that explains in grid format each section. The site is easy to navigate only insofar as the layout is rudimentary and easy to understand – it would be easier to read if the lengthy articles and pages were broken down into manageable chunks. You'll be doing a lot of scrolling: though several pages allow you to jump down to the sections of text you're interested in, you have to scroll back up to get to the navigational strip.

SPECIAL FEATURES

Penis Anatomy and Circumcision The penis 'seems to be one of the most variable elements of the human body in terms of shape and size', as you will discover from this section. There are diagrams detailing the basic anatomy, a lengthy article explaining how it all works, plus several very unerotic pictures of erect and flacid penises. Scroll right down for a piece on circumcision, which is opposed to the practice, and a variety of links, particularly to sites about the foreskin.

Male Sexuality, Arousal and Orgasm is a combination of psychology, biology and sociology, explaining the process of arousal and orgasm, plus related issues such as wet dreams, multiple ejaculations and tantric sex. There are many links to other sex information sites, most of which, like this, are not 'sexy'.

Penis Problems This site covers several of the most common problems associated with penis problems including uridology and gives links to key medical sites that deal with these subjects. Some of the issues addressed are 'frequently asked questions' rather than ailments. The section is divided into six sections: foreskin, glans and shaft problems; other skin problems (such as rashes, bumps and spots); difficulties with size, shape and erection; problems with the testicles and scrotum; sexual issues such as orgasm, premature ejaculation and impotence; and miscellaneous problems (including urinating).

Hypospadias No, we hadn't heard of it either, but incidence of it is apparently increasing. Hypospadias is a condition or 'accident of birth' whereby the opening of the penis (urethral meatus) is found somewhere back along the shaft because the organ has not developed as is most common. It is often accompanied by a hooked appearance and understandably can cause devastating psychological problems. The site strongly recommends and provides links to support groups for the condition (Yahoo has a club). Text in this section provides a definition of hypospadias and why and how it might happen, then considers what can be done about it. Scroll right down and you can read the experiences of site visitors who live with the problem and its most extreme form, epispadias.

Peyronie's differs from hypospadias in that it develops in adult life. The internal tissue of the penis develops into scar tissue and the penis subsequently bends significantly – sometimes dramatically – in a fashion quite different from the curve that is normal in all penises. Some estimate it affects as many as one per cent of men. Psychological problems can develop in turn and in some cases normal intercourse can become impossible. This section is as comprehensive as seems possible because treatment options are currently limited.

Male Menopause is more commonly termed andropause in Europe. It should not be confused with the emotional condition of 'mid-life crisis' which is in humour characterised by the acquisition of a sports car and an 18-year-old girlfriend. Here there is a lengthy piece on mid-life crises backed with expert opinion and comment, but the bulk of this extensive section is on andropause. You can read about one site visitor's personal account of his experience with the condition, which included irritability, irrational behaviour, loss of sex drive, hot flashes, lower back pain, extreme tiredness, plus a vicious circle of depression and impotence. Scroll right down for a lengthy list of typical symptoms and consideration of treatments such as testosterone replacement therapy and Viagra, plus arguments that andropause doesn't really exist. Also here are highly recommended books on the subject.

Links There is a changing selection of recommended sites which, on our last visit, included sites on penis size, enlargement operations, sexual relationships and recommended books. Links are also given throughout the site to relevant pages.

OTHER FEATURES

Penis size, condoms, penis enlargement and other modifications, masturbation and oral sex techniques, female sexuality, gay and bi men.

Sure, there are pictures of penises here, but this information-led site is far from pornographic and rarely crude in its use of language. It deals with emotional issues admirably and will be of particular benefit to young males struggling with questions about normality and safety, older males distressed by changes their bodies and minds are going through as retirement age approaches, and anyone looking to improve their knowledge of the reproductive system or their sexual relations.

www.icr.ac.uk/everyman/
Everyman Action Against Male Cancer

Overall rating: ★ ★ ★ ★

Classification:	Homepage	Readability:	★ ★ ★ ★
Updating:	Varies	Reliability:	★ ★ ★ ★
Navigation:	★ ★ ★ ★	Speed:	★ ★ ★ ★ ★

UK

The homepage of this site reveals that 'Testicular cancer is the most common cancer to affect young men aged between 20–35 years old.' We therefore found it surprising to see that the rest of the homepage is given over to news about what Everyman is doing to combat the illness, rather than information about testicular cancer itself. The theme of promoting the organisation's work is carried throughout the site as it reveals the fund-raising efforts of stars such as Gary Lineker, David Gower, Robbie Williams, and DJ Carl Cox. To navigate the site, choose one of the sections from the menu strip across the top right of the screen, or use one of the quick links to features highlighted on the main part of the screen.

SPECIAL FEATURES

Male Cancers Hidden behind this button, the site provides two online fact sheets, one on testicular cancer, the other on prostate cancer, plus links to cancer patient support organisations and the opportunity to request a copy of the information brochure.

About Everyman explains the campaign and introduces the Everyman centre, which will be the UK's first dedicated male cancer research centre. You can also find out how the campaign's symbol 'the perkin' was created, and take a quiz on male cancers, provided that you have the Flash plug-in.

News and Events Browse the online version of Search, the new Everyman newsletter launched at the tail end of 1999. You can also browse previous editions of the ad hoc Everyman Update newsletter. Here too is the section to check the campaign's events diary, which includes activities ranging from classical and rock music concerts to the Monte Carlo car rally. Alternatively, study their press releases, which seem to be primarily photo opportunities such as 'Scotsmen show us what's really under their kilts to raise awareness of testicular cancer'. However, there are also some chilling research findings in news releases here, for example that over 68 per cent of men aged 15 to 34 know little or nothing about testicular cancer, even though it is the most common cancer amongst young men and rates are doubling every 20 years.

How You Can Help invites visitors to get involved with the fund-raising. You can make a donation, leave a legacy, get your company involved, act as a volunteer, or help fundraise in many other ways.

Press Room offers journalists' biographies of the scientists behind the Everyman campaign, a link to the press releases and a collection of photographs free for press use.

Links to related websites CancerBACUP, the Prostate Cancer Charity, and other sources of cancer and medical information on the internet.

Extremely informative about the campaign, but could do much more to inform visitors about the cancers they aim to raise awareness of. This is a shame, given that the web can be a private medium, one where males can find out about medical matters that they might feel embarrassed to discuss with friends, family or even their doctor.

OTHER SITES OF INTEREST

The Prostate Cancer Charity
www.prostate-cancer.org.uk
Do not be put off by the outdated design – this site is a valuable source of information about prostate cancer. Look here for an explanation of the prostate gland, prostate cancer and the facts regarding diagnosis and treatments. We also found information regarding the possible effect of diet, details of available assistance for sufferers, a list of recommended books and links to related sites.

Men's Health UK
www.menshealth.co.uk
This site exists mainly as promotion for the magazine of the same name, but does offer some editorial tasters. During our visit the selected articles included 'Whacked by the ugly stick', which concerned the common male body flaws women find attractive and 'Press here for great sex' – somewhat self-explanatory! The American edition of Men's

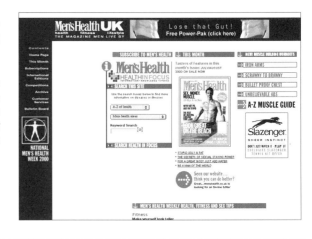

Health has a good site at www.menshealth.com, where you can read articles from the past two years of the magazine.

FHM Bionic
www.fhmbionic.com
Another promotional site for a magazine, but marginally more useful than Men's Health UK. Features include a directory of local gyms, random hangover cures, and a guide to cosmetic surgery for men. You can also check out fatty foods, find out about vitamins and surprise, surprise, learn how to improve your sex life.

Mens Health Tune-Up
http://mens.healthsite.com.au
This attractive Australian site pulls no punches, quoting a random sobering statistic on each page such as 'Depression has been linked with some medical conditions such as cardiovascular disease, diabetes or cancer...' The tune-up is actually a sequence of pages that cover men's health matters such as Cardiovascular Disease, High Blood Pressure, Diabetes, Depression and Arthritis. Choose the 'quick tune-up' option when you arrive on the homepage as this will give you the option of honing in on the subject you're particularly interested in.

Chapter 8

women's health

Most of the major health sites on the internet seem ultimately to be written for women. No matter what the health problem, you can find plenty of useful information in the general medical, complementary therapies and healthy living chapters. The pages here concentrate mainly on sites dedicated to the issues and conditions peculiar to the female body: breasts and the reproductive system.

Their key benefit is not so much in the information they provide, although it's very good, for that is generally widely available on the internet and through other media thanks to women's traditional attentiveness to health matters. Rather, these sites excel at offering support and relieving the sense of isolation that can be experienced by those suffering from reproductive problems and major life changes.

Women's health options have never been greater, or the orthodox approach more controversial. We are freer than ever before to make our own decisions regarding treatments - to follow our medical doctor's favoured course, or to refute it in preference for an alternative method. But with freedom of information comes responsibility to ourselves in researching and assessing it. It is essential to ensure you are fully briefed on arguments for and against the treatments you find discussed on the internet and elsewhere. Make sure you cross-refer to responsible sites offering contrasting opinions, and seek to check information and research findings presented as facts as much as possible. The medical libraries and www.quackwatch.com recommended in the general medical chapter will help in these endeavours.

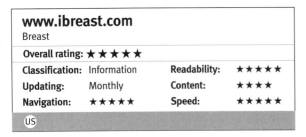

www.ibreast.com
Breast

Overall rating: ★ ★ ★ ★

Classification:	Information	Readability:	★ ★ ★ ★ ★
Updating:	Monthly	Content:	★ ★ ★ ★
Navigation:	★ ★ ★ ★ ★	Speed:	★ ★ ★ ★ ★

US

Your 'complete resource for breast health' is devoted to breast cancer issues. The site is put together by a group of practising physicians and health care professionals, women with breast cancer, researchers, and writers. Founder Dr Marina Weiss was treating breast cancer patients but realised that they had many unmet needs and sought a means of informing and supporting them – the internet was the chosen tool because of its immediacy, interactivity, and ability to override geographical boundaries.

The attractive homepage is easy to navigate, with a 'circle of light' offering information at the left of the screen, certain features highlighted in the centre, and at the right there are links to material from the American Society of Oncologists.

SPECIAL FEATURES

Third Thursday Chats, scheduled to take place at midnight on the third Thursday of each month, aims to help quieten women's nighttime breast cancer fears. At the first chat session, 22 questions from visitors were put to radiation oncologist Dr Weiss. The transcript is featured online.

Prevention talks about the various means of preventing and detecting breast cancer in its early stages, including an illustrated guide to self-examination and discussion of issues surrounding risk factors such as diet and family history. At the right of the screen are links to related pages

entitled 'understanding breast cancer', 'who gets breast cancer', 'breast cancer myths', a piece on tamoxifen (a key drug in treatment), plus a glossary.

Diagnosis includes 'understanding your big picture' to help you assess and understand the 'personality' of your breast cancer – that is, whether it's small and aggressive, large but placid, and so on.

Treatment is divided into articles such as 'understanding your stage', 'surgery', and so on. The features are extensive and detailed but broken down into manageable chunks.

Moving Beyond covers options for reconstructive surgery, how to get on with your life, and understanding menopause.

Recurrence 'We know. This is the last place you wanted to click on,' they say, but information here is hopeful – doctors continue to find new treatments.

Common Ground is designed as a toolkit for understanding and managing the various challenges breast cancer sufferers face on a daily basis – fears, decisions, doctor liaison, planning ahead, enjoying life, and so on.

Resources offers links to recent news stories on breast health, a question and answer facility, recommended books and details of clinical trials.

Links to non-profit associations, US government resources, support organisations, sources of complementary approaches to the disease, news sources.

OTHER FEATURES

Newsletter, event calendar, details of clinical trials, Your Needs survey, quizzes, polls, bulletin boards

A very well-designed site, professionally run, with a great deal of supportive and useful information for British women, even though it is produced by an American team.

www.4woman.org
The National Women's Health Information Center

Overall rating: ★ ★ ★ ★ ★			
Classification:	Information	Readability:	★ ★ ★ ★ ★
Updating:	Daily	Content:	★ ★ ★ ★
Navigation:	★ ★ ★ ★ ★	Speed:	★ ★ ★ ★ ★

US

Produced by the Office on Women's Health at the US Department of Health and Human Services, this site is a lively and intelligent alternative to commercially run women's sites. The homepage offers many points of entry. You can scan the centre of the page for interesting features, but to take it all in, it's easiest to navigate using the left-hand menu panel.

SPECIAL FEATURES

Guest Editor Program sees a person from a nationally-recognised (in the US) magazine contributing an article on a specialised subject. This may be on anorexia, stroke, or endometriosis but, on our last visit, it was 'Your Healthy Pregnancy' by Judith Nolte of American Baby magazine.

Women's Health News Today features reports from Reuters on findings related to women's health – for example the revelation from the US Centers for Disease Control and Prevention that most people using walking as a form of exercise do not walk frequently or fast enough to gain real health benefits, or that a stress hormone has been linked to earlier death in breast cancer sufferers. Also in this section are press releases from the US Department of Health and Human Services, plus details of latest happenings in Congress.

Frequently Asked Questions   Click here and you will be presented with a very large list of topics, from 'acne' to 'weight loss', covering all aspects of women's health plus general health topics such as drug interactions, environmental pollution, health in ethnic populations and a 'ten step countdown to a healthy life'. The answers essentially combine to give a factsheet on each condition, covering what it is, the symptoms, causes, treatments, sources of help and links to specific organisations.

Healthy Pregnancy was a new section on our last visit and a large section in its own right. Move your cursor over the trimesters to see the animated development of the baby in the womb. You can click on each trimester for information on what to expect and what you should do. Altenatively, scroll down and read about family planning, preparing for the new baby, childbirth, after the baby is born, or to take the pregnancy quiz.

Women with Disabilities is a thoughtfully produced channel that aims to recognise that while women with disabilities are women first, they face additional challenges of physical, mental, and sometimes financial limitations. Subjects include abuse, breast health, reproductive health, parenting, sexuality, substance abuse, plus the various types of disability.

Body Image is an educational campaign with handbook that is available to download. Here you will also find tips on nutrition, being active, learning about health, eating disorders and mind-body wellness, with some pages specially for adolescents.

OTHER FEATURES

What's New, Men's Health, For the Media, Health Professionals, Educational Campaigns, Spanish translation.

A tremendous amount of up-to-date and thought-provoking information can be found here.

From the moment the homepage appears, you know this is going to be an excellent resource. It was established in 1996 with the aim of empowering women through health education. The homepage offers many points of entry. Illustrated buttons in the centre of the screen explain the concept and site's facilities – assess, learn, interact, act – and there are two navigational strips; but to get started you should scroll beneath to the Personal Assessments, Health Centers and Personal Services channels.

SPECIAL FEATURES

Personal Assessments offers online quizzes in areas such as reproductive health, menstrual disorders, HRT, midlife sexuality, headaches and depression. You are then presented with information on the subject discussed and links to other pages on the site, such as the FAQ section on that topic.

Health Centers The site offers various 'centers' based on aspects of health such as heart health, midlife (perimenopause and menopause), and depression. They are start-to-finish guides, comprehensive and easy to understand. New at the time of our last visit was the Reproductive Health Center. The Headache Center is sponsored by Glaxo Welcome and affiliated with the American National Headache Foundation. Also here are sections on nutrition, natural health and personal development, the latter being rare amongst health websites and a very positive addition for people that way inclined. As they point out, self-esteem 'is the single most important factor in your health'.

Personal Services has FAQs to read, plus if you register, the opportunity to post questions for various conditions and a 'personal action plan' for helping you manage your health and set and achieve health goals. We did not find this particularly beneficial.

Community Center offers discussion groups and advice, not just on specific health conditions, but the portrayal of women in the media and how to keep a journal. Also here is a mind-body section called Health Convergence, which takes the form of a 'conference' on stress management headed by a women's health psychologist and backed by the results of an online questionnaire.

Research Center is where you can contribute views and experiences to help the site's research - it's not about your attitude to the site itself, but towards women's health subjects and tools such as journaling. The results are used to help institutions such as the Harvard Medical School.

Links to a wide range of women-centred health information services under the Resources Center section. These are divided into specific topics such as behavioural health, cancer, diabetes, endometriosis, osteoporosis, and more.

OTHER FEATURES

News, special events, book sales, polls, newsletter, feedback, US service directory.

The brilliant content suffers a little from the slow speed, but you will enjoy using this well-thought-out and informative site.

www.tidesoflife.com
Goddess Health@Tides of Life

Overall rating: ★ ★ ★ ★

Classification:	Information	Readability:	★ ★ ★ ★
Updating:	Irregular	Content:	★ ★ ★ ★
Navigation:	★ ★ ★	Speed:	★ ★ ★

US

A stunning picture of The Goddess of Tides emerging from the waves in a cute frock is the inspiring choice of illustration for this site's homepage. Few of us feel like that while experiencing PMS or menopause, but the message here is that one can 'emerge victoriously' from the problems associated with the female reproductive cycle when one turns to natural, drug-free therapies.

The design of the site is rather old fashioned. You need to scroll down quite a long way to get a measure of what is here and you will either take to it immediately or not as the approach is not only holistic but very alternative. 'This is not mainstream information,' they warn us while emphasising that the mission is to provide 'current, relevant information from many sources'.

Suggested Reading The books recommended on the homepage are a good indication of the style of information preferred here: *The Estrogen Alternative*, *Women's Bodies Women's Wisdom* and *The Menopause Industry: How the Medical Establishment Exploits Women* are key titles.

The Library Here you will find a long list of articles divided into general categories including PMS, Menopause and Anti-aging, ERT and HRT Information, Pregnancy and Fertility Issues, and miscellaneous women's health information, including a piece arguing that sex can be better after menopause, and the debate about a link between dietary fat and breast cancer. There is also an extended recommended reading list. Typical features are 'herbs to use and avoid in pregnancy', 'depression, obesity and herbal remedies', and 'taking the mystery out of menstruation'.

Referrals While British readers will not generally be needing to find alternative therapists in the US, this section is worth a look for its advice on making the decision to use complementary and alternative therapies. It looks at safety issues, how to establish the expertise of a practitioner, how to assess the service and cost. An important point is that the site aims to help you enlist the support of your doctor in exploring natural therapies.

OTHER FEATURES

Photo gallery, natural 'be good to your man' section, sales.

For those women who like to think outside the box on health matters, this site will prove interesting and inspiring, if controversial.

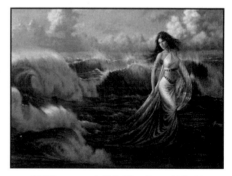

Goddess of the Tides

PMS & Menopause can be like the Tides. Emerge victoriously!

www.menopause.net
Menopause.net

Overall rating: ★ ★ ★ ★

Classification:	Information	Readability:	★ ★ ★ ★ ★
Updating:	Infrequently	Content:	★ ★ ★ ★
Navigation:	★ ★ ★ ★ ★	Speed:	★ ★ ★ ★ ★

US

This site is sponsored by Organon, a medicine research and development company that to date has specialised in the fields of hormone research and gynaecology. While this is worth knowing, the company's promotion on the site is very unobtrusive and the content, while medically-oriented, is geared towards education about menopause rather than selling drugs to alleviate the symptoms. It does, however, frequently suggest you speak to your doctor about HRT.

The homepage is a little old fashioned in design and uses frames but is easy to understand and navigate. It does not give the impression that it is jam-packed with useful information, but there is a great deal here once you start browsing the articles. There are two menus, one down either side of the page. The left-hand side concentrates on introductory fact sheets and general information, while the right-hand menu looks at body-specifics.

SPECIAL FEATURES

Needs explains the short and long term issues women facing menopause are likely to encounter and reveals the physical and emotional challenges typically faced at each stage of the process. It also introduces the reader to HRT (hormone replacement therapy), briefly outlining the pros and cons.

Well-Being   There are some women who sail through menopause barely batting an eyelid. Others experience the nagging symptoms outlined here. Vasomotor symptoms are the hot flushes and night sweats, then there are mood issues such as irritability, poor memory and lack of concentration, and problems with libido and sexuality. This section is reassuring in its tone – no, you're not the only one as statistics show – and offers practical tips for alleviating symptoms.

Bone moves from menopause into the related condition of osteoporosis. Here you can learn the basics of bone health, facts about osteoporosis, how to 'invest' in your bones (give up smoking, don't get drunk a lot, be active, eat calcium and, of course, consider HRT!) and take a quick yes-or-no osteoporosis risk quiz.

Endometrium looks at issues surrounding menopause, monthly periods and HRT. As the site points out, one of the few advantages of menopause is that you no longer have periods, so it's no wonder many women refuse to take HRT treatments that cause the periods to continue.

Cardiovascular is not about cardio exercise, but cardiovascular disease and the fact that the risk of it suddenly increases in postmenopausal women. It's a myth that only men suffer with heart problems, and this section looks at lifestyle habits you can adopt as well as a balanced assessment of the role HRT may play.

Urogenital Complaints of this nature increase substanitally with age and, while symptoms may not develop until several years after menopause, they are related to the loss of oestrogen. Expect therefore vaginal dryness and problems with urinary function, but find out how to cope with them here.

Breast As this site confirms, a major concern of women is the possible link between breast cancer and HRT. This section is important to read as it features a great deal of information on the controversy and admits that nagging breast tenderness is another unpleasant side effect of HRT.

Links There are some, but it is not a comprehensive range of other reference sources.

OTHER FEATURES

More on HRT, general info, fact sheet, common questions, glossary

A better site would consider natural remedies as well as HRT. However, there are plenty of tips given here regarding lifestyle changes ('take frequent, lukewarm showers', 'reduce caffeine consumption', and so on) that will be beneficial to those visitors entering menopause. It is an excellent source of information for those new to the subject.

www.dearest.com
Power Surge

Overall rating: ★ ★ ★ ★			
Classification:	Information	**Readability:**	★ ★ ★ ★
Updating:	Weekly	**Content:**	★ ★ ★ ★
Navigation:	★ ★ ★	**Speed:**	★ ★ ★

US

An impressive sequence of Flash-based animation set to a thriving disco beat is the exciting opener to this long-running site which claims to be the number one menopause support group on the internet. It's enough to make you feel as though menopause is the most glamorous thing that could ever happen to you and no doubt brings tears to the eyes of many sufferers. The 'Dearest' referred to throughout the site was the online persona of the site's founder Alice Lotto Stamm, who came up with the phrase Power Surge to describe her experience of hot flushes.

Sit back (unless you feel like dancing) until the homepage appears. A scrolling list of timely and interesting points is presented under the Newsworthy heading at the left of the screen. A menu button is situated at the top right. Click on it and a box will appear from which you can choose a department. Most of the articles are contained under Transcripts. The site is difficult to navigate – click on Library and you find yourself in Transcripts.

SPECIAL FEATURES

Guest Conferences You can find out about these in advance by choosing Schedule from the menu box. There is an impressive list of doctors, PhDs and authors, covering a variety of menopause-related topics such as weight loss, heart health, soy protein, female sexuality, and – curiously

– magic movie moments. Many of the guests are TV stars in the US, which adds a frisson for American site visitors. You can view the transcripts of previous sessions by choosing the Transcripts link from the main menu box.

Web Chats are also featured at America Online, a key supporter of Dearest. The open dialogues take place every Thursday at 9pm (US ET) and cover aspects of menopause such as simple ways to cope with depression, loss of libido, and so on.

Message Boards are divided into a long list of individual subjects and are very well attended.

Ask the Experts Click here and you will be presented with a series of search boxes for questions answered previously by the doctor, weight-loss expert, relationship expert, and the medical director of the soy protein product manufacturer. Unfortunately, the archive is arranged by date and not subject. This section was badly organised: what exactly would be a good keyword to type in for weight loss for example? Fat? Thin? Diet? And we were unimpressed with the brevity of the answers.

Reading Room is also referred to as the Power Surge Resource Center. There is a fair amount of crossover here with other sections, but you will find links, recommended products, access to transcripts and chat plus a quick-reference HRT brand-dose chart.

OTHER FEATURES

Weekly poll, books, recommended product suppliers, newsletters.

Although more commercial in its approach than other sites (makers of soy protein are sponsors), this is a welcoming and lively source of information and support for those dealing with menopause issues. It's a pity the information is so disorganised.

OTHER SITES OF INTEREST

MUM: the Museum of Menstruation and Women's Health
www.mum.org
A multi-award winning site curiously put together by a man, Harry Finley. The homepage's background illustration is derived from an old tampon box and content ranges from serious to amusing and lewd. Look here should you want to find out more about menstruation history, what religions have had to say on the subject, practical issues such as the safety of menstrual products, or if you want a laugh.

Women Central
www.women.com
This general women's site has a health and wellness channel nestled in amongst the horoscopes, book and movie reviews. It works in conjunction with respected American magazines such as Prevention and Redbook and covers lifestyle, alternative medicine, medical conditions, family health and aging. There a plenty of articles plus a range of tools, quizzes and calculators. The team here also supplies the editorial content to Microsoft's women's channel (womencentral.msn.com), which features several lively health articles on a weekly basis.

Menstruation.com.au
www.menstruation.com.au
If you are looking to turn your monthly cycle into a celebratory spiritual experience, this is the site for you. It intriguingly combines astrology, natural fertility, lunar phases and yoga with discussion of PMS and organic tampons.

Breakthrough Breast Cancer
www.breakthrough.org.uk

This highly successful charity has played a major role in raising the awareness of and funding research into breast cancer in the UK, including the British arm of the trendy Fashion Targets Breast Cancer appeal. The beautifully designed site concentrates not on information about the disease but how you can support the organisation and help raise money for the fight against breast cancer.

PCOS.net
www.pcos.net

The aim of this site is to provide information and support for women with polycustic ovarian syndrome, one of the main causes of infertility and yet a problem that is very difficult to diagnose. The pages are put together by two sufferers but managed on a reasonably professional level. You will find details of research studies and support groups. As with so many things in life, the symptoms of PCOS are relieved by achieving a sensible weight, so the low-carbohydrate diet generally used in managing symptoms is a key part of the site, although they recommend several specific eating plans.

Kotex
www.uk.kotex.com

The site of the British arm of this international sanitary protection company is more groovy than its American sister, which has a naff picture of a girl rollerblading on its homepage. The UK version is designed to look like a scrapbook and is aimed at teenagers who need to learn more about the products available and the challenges associated with menstruation, such as PMS, mood swings, and going to the gynaecologist. There is also 'Girlthing', a magazine-style section with lifestyle advice, message boards, quizzes and so on.

Menopause Online
www.menopause-online.com

There is a friendly, personal tone to this natural-remedy led site on menopause. You can contribute to the 13 or so message boards which cover topics such as meditation, sleeping problems, irregular bleeding, anxiety/depression and surgery. There are poems, cartoons and a column from Emily, a sufferer, plus news and coverage of scientific studies.

The North American Menopause Society
www.menopause.org

The NMAS claims to be the leading nonprofit scientific organisation devoted to menopause. The easy-to-navigate site includes pages for the general public and health professionals. A key concern of the organisation is to publish consensus opinions on clinical issues – sadly, these are not myriad when it comes to menopause.

Chapter 9

children's health

A few of the sites recommended here are written and designed especially for children, however for the most part this chapter focuses on sites with information about children's health for parents. Baby and parenting sites are amongst the most popular and high profile sites on the web - due in part no doubt to the ecommerce opportunities they provide for the owners and publishers who are prepared to advertise them heavily. But there are other reasons: parents are often more anxious about the health of their children than they are about their own, and first-timers naturally want to learn as much as they can in order to produce and raise children to the best of their ability.

The interactivity of the internet adds an element of fun to these sites with several offering calculators and analysing tools to help you estimate date, size and even sex. More

seriously, you can learn how to make a birth plan to help everything run as smoothly as possible and the way you want it to.

Many of the general baby and parenting sites deal with the subject from pre-conception to schooling, so they are also good points of reference for couples trying or even struggling to become parents. Traditional medical advice is covered, but also psychological and behavioural issues, and there is plenty of advice and instruction on self-care and first aid for minor problems that don't require the attention of a doctor. Anyone trying or getting ready to have a baby should also take a look at the sites dedicated to the process of childbirth, for today's parents-to-be have myriad choices when it comes to delivery and complex decisions to make. It's enough to turn anyone into an information junkie.

www.babyworld.co.uk
Babyworld

Overall rating: ★ ★ ★ ★ ★			
Classification:	Information	**Readability:**	★ ★ ★ ★ ★
Updating:	Daily	**Content:**	★ ★ ★ ★ ★
Navigation:	★ ★ ★ ★	**Speed:**	★ ★ ★

UK

Babyworld was started by a medical publisher based in Oxford, but was famously bought out by Freeserve, the internet service provider. The homepage looks rather like a traditional magazine cover, with a large picture of a happy baby and various features highlighted around him. The channels are listed in a menu panel of buttons that takes rather a long time to appear down the left-hand side of the screen. Membership is required to enter competitions, giveaways and access the member services area, which includes the community facilities, an online antenatal club and other tools.

SPECIAL FEATURES

News & Features includes new products on the market as well as news-based articles, such as the launch of a new vaccine or coverage of a new report from a children's organisation or charity. Our last visit saw them expanding on the decision of Britain's first gay fathers of surrogate twins to try for a third child – a saga the site had already been covering in some depth. Archived stories and product reviews are available.

Trying for a Baby is divided into two main sections: 'essential information' on how to maximise your chances of becoming pregnant, and 'for dads', which raises issues such as paternity leave, sex in pregnancy, whether to attend the birth and what to take to it.

Pregnancy has plenty of useful information for those who are not yet pregnant, such as a timeline of what you need to do and what to expect, advice on eating, working, and exercise during pregnancy, useful books, and much more.

Birth The 'essential information' section of this channel reveals what happens in labour, how to make a birth plan, types of pain relief for labour, types of birth, how to change your GP or midwife, support organisations, and plenty of other reference information.

Your Baby offers an A–Z of child health, tips on telling when s/he is ill, and homeopathic remedies for babies. Essential information includes a developmental chart, advice on holding, handling and feeding, changing nappies and bathing, and what you need to know about babies crying.

New Parents What to do about returning to work and childcare options, plus money and legal assistance, are topics covered here.

Ask our Experts A doctor, midwife, breastfeeding expert and fertility expert are available to answer your questions, but you need to check the site first to make sure the query has not been answered already. 'It is one of Baby World's top priorities to try to provide an answer to every member's question, whatever aspect of parenting it concerns,' they state. Answers to frequently asked questions are accessed by clicking on the bottom at the right of the screen – you will then be given a choice of subject areas in a pull-down menu.

OTHER FEATURES

Shopping, product testing, recipes, recommended books, community.

If you have a question that the site has not already answered we'd be surprised. This is a comprehensive and useful information resource, as well as a good opportunity to make contact with other parents and parents-to-be.

www.kidshealth.org
Kids Health

Overall rating: ★ ★ ★ ★ ★			
Classification:	Information	Readability:	★ ★ ★ ★ ★
Updating:	Weekly	Content:	★ ★ ★ ★ ★
Navigation:	★ ★ ★ ★ ★	Speed:	★ ★ ★ ★

US

The organisation behind this site is the Nemours Foundation, a nonprofit group and 'the largest physician practice delivering subspecialty pediatric care in the United States'. Unlike other sites associated with children and health, this one has channels for the kids rather than about them. The homepage is divided into three main sections, one for each age group, and you simply need to click on the entry button for the area you are interested in. The latest features added to each section are highlighted on the homepage. Once inside a channel you can search the site by keyword.

SPECIAL FEATURES

Parents offers a tip of the day to do with kids' health and a featured article. Click on the What's New button to find out the latest additions to the site which, on our last visit included articles on childhood depression, sun safety and common surgeries for kids. The main menu of reference articles is listed down the right half of the screen and offers general advice on health and caring for your child, plus sections dedicated to infections, emotions and behaviour, growth and development, nutrition and fitness, pregnancy and newborns, first aid and safety. Positive Parenting offers advice on issues such as homework, discipline and how to talk to your child about sex, tobacco and alcohol. Look under Medical Problems for features such as 'managing asthma',

'when your child has cerebral palsy', 'when your baby is born with a health problem', and 'kidney diseases in childhood' – there are an admirable number of topics covered in sensitive and reassuring fashion This channel also offers weekly news analysis – the staff report on the most recent advances in children's health and aim to keep you posted on research which may affect you and your child.

Kids can be very slow to load, unlike the parents channel. This is divided into several sections to educate children about their growing bodies and looking after them, to help them understand illness, hospitals, and so on. There is a glossary-cum-dictionary, healthy recipes, games and pages dedicated to dealing with feelings and emotional issues such as friendship. It's fun, educational and well illustrated.

Teens New features for teenagers on our most recent visit were a guide to the reproductive system, the risk of getting pregnant while menstruating, dietary supplements 'Facts vs Fads', and tips for healthy travel. There is the opportunity to send questions in for answering, plus a category devoted to healthy eating, recipes, sports and eating disorders.

OTHER FEATURES

Email newsletters.

A very well-designed site with authoritative age-appropriate content that is very easy to understand. Kids Health is sure to be of help when children are sick – whether it is you visiting the site, or them.

www.iparenting.com
iParenting

Overall rating: ★ ★ ★ ★ ★			
Classification:	Information	**Readability:**	★ ★ ★ ★ ★
Updating:	Daily	**Content:**	★ ★ ★ ★ ★
Navigation:	★ ★ ★ ★ ★	**Speed:**	★ ★ ★ ★

US

iParenting is a group of 17 websites devoted to families from preconception through to teenage years. It was founded by the 'webmother' Elisa Ast All and her husband Alvin in 1996 after she concluded that expectant and new parents were underserved on the internet – a situation certainly no longer apparent. You can access all the sites from this one URL; however, it is the umbrella for a variety including Preconception.com, BabiesToday.com, Breastfeed.com and TeenagersToday.com as well as subsites such as BirthStories.com and CycleDaily.com, which has pages on fertility. The company has been so successful it has expanded into 'lifestyle' sites including RecipesToday.com.

The network is very easy to navigate and clear, despite the cutesy 'handwriting' of headlines and buttons. The main menu panel is down the left-hand side of the screen with the news and interactive elements featured in a box on the right.

SPECIAL FEATURES

Breastfeed You can breastfeed and still have it all, we were told on our last visit, whether 'all' of it is a cup of coffee in the morning, a beer with your spicy Mexican dinner, or a cold remedy. This site advises on the lifestyle of breast feeding as well as Q&A with experts and sharing of reader diaries.

Preschoolers Today, 'celebrating ages three, four and five', deals largely with behavioural and educational issues. There are some good tips on educational play, such as taking your kid into the garden to help explain why beans don't actually come from the grocery store.

Preteenagers Today is for parents of kids aged 10–12. Typical content deals with what you should do if your child believes the whole world hates her, or is telling lies a great deal. An interesting question asked of contributing expert child psychologist Tracy Underwood was, 'Are my kids being overstimulated with so many extra-curricular activities?'

Resources and Tools Dr William Sears and his wife Martha, who is a registered nurse and author of 25 Things Every New Mother Should Know, write articles and answer questions from site visitors in this section. There is an index of answers to previous questions and, to help with research, you can search the section by keyword. Also here are regular articles by the site's founder and editor-in-chief Elisa Ast All.

Dads Today 'Webfather' Alvin hosts this section offering up-to-date news and expert Q&A dealing with relationships, behaviour, discipline, safety and money management. Other dads pitch in, too, through reader diaries and discussion groups, including the tip to wear a protective cup to the delivery room in case a wife in the throes of labour tries to rip off his manhood in revenge.

Links to websites relevant to feature articles, such as identifying poisonous plants.

OTHER FEATURES

News, book and video reviews and sales, Spanish version, plus the various other sites in the network.

iParenting is an essential reference for parents aiming to deal with behavioural and psychological issues. The tone is welcoming, supportive and positive, but if you're looking for medical information specific to children, this is not the place to be.

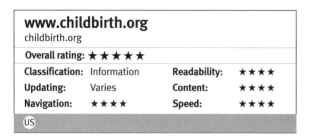

www.childbirth.org
childbirth.org

Overall rating: ★ ★ ★ ★ ★			
Classification:	Information	**Readability:**	★ ★ ★ ★
Updating:	Varies	**Content:**	★ ★ ★ ★
Navigation:	★ ★ ★ ★	**Speed:**	★ ★ ★ ★

US

'Birth is a natural process, not a medical procedure' is the slogan of this long-running site produced by a group of childbirth professionals including midwives, nurses and doulas. The homepage presents a long list of departments in a menu panel down the left-hand side of the screen. New additions to the site are highlighted underneath the welcome at the centre of the page and immediately below is a keyword search facility.

SPECIAL FEATURES

Ask the Pros is divided into sections according to the type of expert – childbirth educator, doula, fitness pro, lactation consultant, midwife, nurse – many more types of specialists than normally featured on this type of section. You can submit your own question and, of course, view previous responses.

Birth Plans are a written statement about your preferences for labour and birth. In this section there are links to pages on birth plans covering FAQs, legal ramifications, choices available and how they may later affect breastfeeding, plus an interactive online birth plan. Beneath are several examples of real life birth plans from site visitors and the opportunity to contribute your own.

Birth Stories seem to be a popular feature of parenting sites. Childbirth.org handles it well by pointing out right away that

these are experiences of the general public and the views they may express are not professional medical opinion. The birth stories are categorised into small batches for leisure reading, or by theme, and you can contribute your own.

Girl or Boy is an interactive quiz that determines your baby's gender based on old wives' tales. It's just a fun load of tosh, not a guarantee of outcome.

Caesareans features many links of interest to people who expect to or have given birth by Caesarean section. It includes several FAQs plus a video, a history, advice on breastfeeding after the birth, and switching to vaginal birth on the next occasion, plus lots more.

Complications Heaven forbid; however, this section features advice on how to identify and deal with complications that may arise during pregnancy, labour and birth. There are several types of complication listed for each category, so reading here is a must for mums-to-be.

Links to About.com, Amazon, Health A-Z, Baby Universe, plus many specialist web pages.

OTHER FEATURES

Several more categories of childbirth information, plus book sales, postcards, class finder, birth stories, newsletter and competitions.

What this site lacks in design it makes up for in comprehensive coverage. You will particularly enjoy this site if you are looking for health advice that is empowering and emotionally supportive rather than just medically accurate.

www.parents.com

Parents.com

Overall rating: ★ ★ ★

Classification:	Ezine	Readability:	★ ★ ★ ★
Updating:	Varies	Content:	★ ★ ★ ★
Navigation:	★ ★ ★ ★	Speed:	★ ★ ★ ★

US

Parents.com is a site built on extracts from leading American women's magazines including Child, Parents and Family Circle. Given this, it's surprising the site is so unattractive and, at first glance, seems to contain little. A look at the site map, however, reveals that there is a great deal of content here. Some features are highlighted on the uninspiring homepage. Choose a channel from the blue menu strip at the top of the screen and you will be transported to a page offering many more relevant choices. There are two search facilities at the top of the page - one based on keywords and the other on pulldown menus for subject and age group, though the pulldown menu facility did not work well.

SPECIAL FEATURES

Pregnancy Some of this content is a little girly, frankly, but that's no surprise given that it comes from popular women's magazines. Amongst the articles are a guide to the normal progress of pregnancy through the trimesters, information on labour, delivery and postpartum, a 'new parent survival guide' including supplies, know-how and tips for mum and dad, plus an ask the (ob-gyn) expert section.

Health and Safety This channel is the highlight of the site and contains advice not so prominent on other parenting web resources. Here you will find essential information on maximising the safety of your children in the home, at playtime, when out and about, plus advice on problem

prevention and treatment. In line with other websites there is a product recall warning section relevant to the US market. You can also ask questions of the site's paediatrician. Typical features include tips on making sure your pool is safe for children, situations where it may be okay for kids to go barefoot, how to establish the safety of fireworks, bicycle seats, and so on.

Development covers the growth of the child from birth onwards. Each age bracket is divided into physical, cognitive, emotional and social development. As the child gets older, behaviour and discipline are also covered. Useful were the features 'Ten Discipline Lessons to Live By', how to prevent learning loss during the long summer holidays, and how to establish whether or not you are spoiling your child.

Living discusses issues such as child care, working parents, education, children and the media, family life, finances and recommended books on these subjects.

Fun suggests various different types of books, movies and videos, music, television, software and websites, toys and games and parties for children. There are some great ideas, such as the recipe for homemade play dough and ideas for themed kids' parties.

Ask the Expert includes a nutritionist and 'travel mom' as well as healthcare professionals. Biographies of each expert are provided and questions are answered within two weeks, if at all. They aim to make those posted queries answered representative of what most visitors have been asking.

OTHER FEATURES

Food, travel, shopping

If you don't mind ignoring the information that is relevant only to Americans, this is a useful and inspiring site for young parents to visit.

www.webbaby.co.uk
Web Baby

Overall rating: ★ ★ ★ ★			
Classification:	Information	**Readability:**	★ ★ ★ ★
Updating:	Monthly	**Reliability:**	★ ★ ★ ★
Navigation:	★ ★ ★	**Speed:**	★ ★ ★ ★

UK

Web Baby is the brainchild of Kirsty Oliver, a chartered accountant, and Gill Thorn, an antenatal teacher. The site has an advisory board including doctors specialising in paediatrics, obstetrics and gynaecology. Shopping is a key element – and some of the advertised products are highly desirable – but this is primarily an information and community URL. If you register you can get a ten percent discount in the baby boutique.

The site looks reasonably attractive and is easy to understand; however, it is plodding to navigate as the material is broken down into so many subcategories. The main menu panel is down the left of the screen with some features highlighted at centre.

SPECIAL FEATURES

Preconception There are loads of useful things you could be doing to aid yourself in getting pregnant – apart from the obvious. This section covers fertility problems, antenatal health, new products and ideas, preconception care, fitness and nutrition, and, believe it or not, a mobile phone service that will send you reminders of your most fertile period. Amongst the interactive tools are an ovulation calculator, pre-baby weight calculator, chromosome abnormality calculator, and a due date calculator.

Pregnancy 'What to eat, drink, wear, how to sleep, get rid of heartburn and hide the bags under your eyes.' Also here are the details of your baby's progress in the womb and insight into the hospital tests and visits you will be undertaking.

Baby features issues you will face once the baby arrives, and health is obviously a key element. Immunisation, bottlefeeding, development, breast feeding, crying, colic, and child psychology are amongst the subjects included.

Toddler is very similar to the above section, but brings in issues for older children such as education, and what to do with a fussy eater.

Dr Web's Clinic re-presents the database of articles in another format, which is surprising because this seemed like a more interactive feature given the channel's strapline: 'Medical Advice Online'. There is a large button to the top right of the screen which you can click to peruse the online clinic schedule.

Community aims to break through the isolation that is felt by many parents-to-be and young mums. You need to register with Web Baby to use the chat rooms and post messages on the boards. They do not seem to be well attended, sadly.

WebBaby Directory provides contact details for a wide range of organisations and helplines around the UK and these are divided into subject category.

OTHER FEATURES

Shopping, online photo album, gift registry, newsletter, tips on playing with baby, what's new, press releases.

It's an editorial challenge, breaking down so much information into manageable chunks; however, moving through the various subcategories of each subject to try and actually read some information feels rather like jumping through hoops, which is a shame because the information here is good.

OTHER SITES OF INTEREST

The Adventures of Mr Reach
www.jnjoralhealth.com
Produced by Johnson and Johnson, this is an exellent site for helping you to teach children to brush their teeth. There are separate sections for parents and children, plus Mr Reach's Toolbox, which is a guide to dental hygiene products.

The Miscarriage Association
www.the-ma.org.uk
'Acknowledging pregnancy loss' is the aim of this British association. As the homepage quotes: 'When I lost my baby they said it happens to one in four pregnancies. But when I came out of hospital there was no one to talk to.' The site works on frames and is a little fiddly to view on a small screen, but navigation is relatively straightforward. They concentrate on explaining what services are available from the organisation rather than offering the services online, but you can read back issues of the quarterly newsletter and browse the recommended links.

Child: the National Infertility Support Network
www.child.org.uk
This site, like the organisation, aims to provide high quality information and support to those suffering from infertility, as well as to promote public awareness of the problem and its impact on the quality of life of those who suffer from it. Here you can peruse articles on infertility and related issues, several of which are taken from BBC News Online. Unfortunately, the interactive facilities are not up to par; there are no forums or chat rooms, which may be one of the most effective means of achieving their stated aim of helping to eradicate the isolation felt by couples with infertility problems. However, there is an excellent annotated links section.

I Wanna Know
www.iwannaknow.org
Regardless of your views about the site's misguided attempt to be right-on through poor spelling, I Wanna Know is an admirable attempt to supply teenagers with responsible information regarding sexual health and relationships. It covers the basics of puberty, plus sexually transmitted diseases and sexual orientation. There are chat rooms and a section for concerned parents too.

International Planned Parenthood Federation
www.ippf.org
The IPPF is a voluntary organisation focusing on sexual and reproductive health, plus family planning, and is active in more than 180 countries worldwide. Working in conjunction with the BBC World Service, it has recently launched the Sexwise radio series in eleven languages to reach 60 million listeners in areas such as Africa, the Arab world, Latin America, China and Southeast Asia. Here you can learn more about the organisation's activities and publications in the field of reproductive rights and teen sex education.

BrainPOP
www.brainpop.com
In its entirety this cute site has more than 80 original animated movies on health, science and technology for children. The aim is to answer common kids' questions about their bodies and how they work. Click on the health movie button to be taken through to the illustrated menu (unfortunately slow to load). Specific topics include the biology-related homeostasis, cells, blood, nerve, and brain, lifestyle health subjects including fitness and nutrition, plus specific conditions such as diabetes, lyme disease, cancer and, more widespread, acne. You may find this site useful when it comes to explaining menstruation too.

Fertile Thoughts
www.fertilethoughts.net
The homepage of this site dealing with infertility, adoption and subsequent parenting issues is attractively illustrated but unfortunately very slow to load. The channels appear in a circle around the main logo, giving the impression that there is not much content, and at the time of our review much of the content was 'coming soon...'. Navigation is a little tricky: once you are in the channel, you need to click on the top section of the white menu strip to choose a section and then pick the desired pages from the pink menu strip immediately underneath. The text in the main section of the screen won't change until you do this. The Infertility channel has interactive facilities such as forums on endometriosis, living childfree, IVF treatment, miscarriage and trying to conceive after a loss, and a 'be informed' section that includes a good 'ask the doctor' facility and the ability to search by keyword for previous answers.

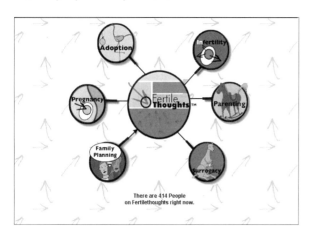

index